SYSTEMA INSTRUCTOR

Robert Poyton

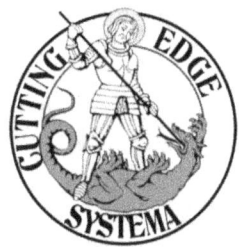

Copyright@ 2022 R Poyton

All rights reserved

The moral right of the author has been asserted

No part of this book may be reproduced in any form or by any
electronic or mechanical means including information storage
and retrieval systems, without permission in writing from the author.
The only exception is by a reviewer, who may quote short
excerpts in a review.

The author and publisher take no responsibility for any illness or
injury resulting from practicing the exercises described in this book.
Always consult your Doctor prior to training or if you have any medical issues.

Published by Cutting Edge

978-1-7399855-7-8

"I know that you believe you understand what you think I said, but I am not sure you realize that what you heard is not what I meant!"
- Quote from a U.S. government official

ABOUT THE AUTHOR

Robert was born in the early 1960's in East London. He trained in Judo and boxing as a child and at age 18 began training in Yang Family Taijiquan.

For many years he studied the Chinese Internal Arts in depth. In the 1990's he set up his own school and began cross training in several styles.

In 2000 he began training in Systema and has since trained extensively with with Mikhail Ryabko and Vladimir Vasiliev in both Moscow and Toronto. In addition he has arranged numerous UK seminars for Mikhail, Vladimir and other instructors.

Robert now trains solely in Systema and runs regular classes in the UK and teaches seminars throughout the UK and Europe. He has been featured in numerous martial arts books and magazines as well as producing his own publications and training films.

Outside of training, Robert is a professional musician and currently lives in rural Bedfordshire with his wife and a small menagerie.

"Rob Poyton has been training and teaching Systema since 2000. He is a dedicated and talented instructor, knowledgeable on all of the key components of Systema. Rob presents his teaching in a clear and structured manner through his classes and reading materials."
- Vladimir Vasiliev, October 2019.

*Dedicated to my teachers
Mikhail and Vladimir,
and to everyone I ever trained
with or taught.*

Thank you.

CONTENTS

CHAPTER 1: INTRODUCTION
Martial Arts Types 9
What is Systema? 11

CHAPTER 2: FIRST STEPS
Why Teach? 15

CHAPTER 3: SETTING UP A CLASS
Venues 21
Paperwork 25
Promotion 26
Social Media 29
Presentation 32

CHAPTER 4: RUNNING A CLASS
Formality 35
Motivation 36
Consent 41
Fees 46
Equipment 49
Class Types 50

CHAPTER 5: CLASS STRUCTURE
Lesson Plans 59
How Much to Explain? 62
Pacing a Class 65
What to Teach? 66

CHAPTER 6: MANAGING A CLASS
Learning Styles 73
Mutual Benefit 77
Relax! 83
Intensity 85
Mindset 88
Flow State 90
Challenges 92
Emotions 100

CHAPTER 7: DRILLS AND EXERCISES
Exercises 109
Drills 110
The Four Pillars 112
Time Slices 115
Ten Points of Sparring 120
Technique or Principle? 131
Creating Drills 132

CHAPTER 8: CLASS CONTENT
Fundamentals 137
Integration 145
Refinement 148
Testing 153
Creating Fear 163

CHAPTER 9: WORKSHOPS
In House 169
Hosting 175
Courses 177
Camps 179
Instructor Training 185

CHAPTER 10: CONCLUSIONS
Future Development 188

APPENDICES
Class Notes 193
Waiver Examples 197
7 Principles of Breathing 199
9 Requirements of Flow 201
Camp Information Example 203
How to be a Good Student 205

CHAPTER ONE
INTRODUCTION

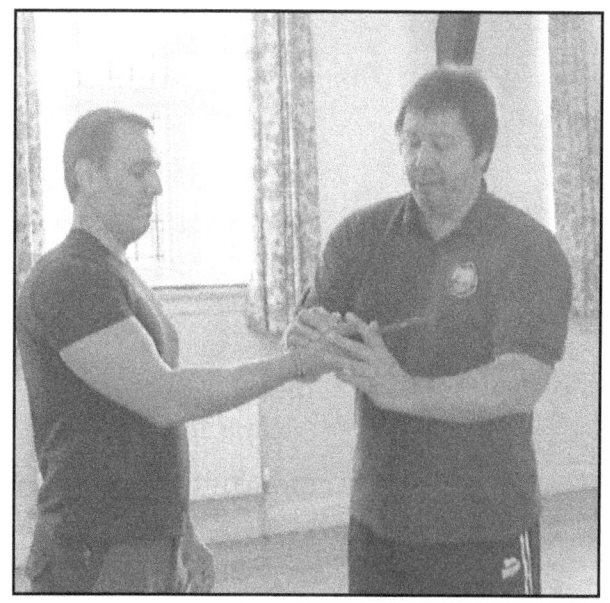

While Systema has deep roots, both in terms of history and practice, it is a relatively recent newcomer to the martial arts mainstream. Most people are used to the ideas and general concepts of the various forms of Karate, Kung Fu, Judo and so on. They might also have some exposure to modern combative systems such as Krav Maga, as well as combat sports like BJJ, MMA and so on. However, despite its rapid growth over the last twenty years, most people outside of martial arts have not heard of Systema. And those inside martial arts may well have polarised views about it, largely based on negative social media posts.

If we look at the above, we see that we can broadly divide martial arts into four categories:

Traditional - an emphasis on set routines, a highly structured syllabus, often a grading system, an established lineage dating back to the founders of the art, cultural / aesthetic traditions, a health / meditation component, students often wear a particular outfit or uniform, classes tend to be formal.

Combatives - a set number of easy to learn techniques, emphasis on speed and aggression, pressure and scenario training, occasional grading system, emphasis on civilian or military self defence.

Combat sports - techniques specific to a rule set, emphasis on fitness, opportunity to compete, less emphasis on style, culture or art.

Synthesis arts - attempts to blend various styles together to cover all aspects of combat. For example, Jeet Kune Do, Bruce Lee's art (blending Chinese styles and concepts with Western boxing, fencing, etc), less focus on lineage and tradition, more focus on direct application

These are general observations, of course there are cross-overs and exceptions. But overall most styles fit neatly into one of those categories. And this is where some have problems understanding what Systema is.

Like many, on first encounter I viewed it as a form of military combatives. The first video I saw (the TRS *Red Zone* series) framed much of its advertising and content in military / professional terms. In fact, a lot of that initial material had the same feel, this was all very direct, combatives-type work.

There were also a number of current and ex military training in Systema, so it seemed natural to peg it as "combatives." However, even at that time, there were practices and references to deeper material. The very first time I trained with Vladimir, around 2000, he was talking about massage and breath-work, for example. He also showed a range of shoulder and spinal manipulation exercises. This only served to pique my interest even further.

At the time I had a considerable background in traditional Chinese martial arts, which included various methods of qigong, massage, medicine and so on. However these, like many aspects of those arts, were set in a cultural tradition that could be somewhat opaque at times. So, then, Systema was not just "combatives," it was a traditional martial art!

Well, no... at least not in the sense I was used to. No gradings (though to be fair, very few "old school" Chinese styles have gradings), no uniform, no bowing or formality (everyone shakes hands, there are no titles of honorifics), no kata or forms to memorise, no stories of the feats of masters from long ago. Most of all, none of those cultural trappings in terms of clothing, terminology or concepts.

So not a traditional art, then! But hang on - there's a wealth of work on health, well-being, internal work, emotional and psychological balancing, and an underlying spirituality, with its roots in the Orthodox Christian church. Okay, so now I'm confused!

Ah, but surely we can all agree on the fact that Systema is not useful for combat sports? Yet I've trained with and trained experienced wrestlers, Thai boxers, BJJ people, boxers and so on. The puzzle deepens!

That only leaves synthesis arts. Surely this must be the one! Systema incorporates ground work, punches, kicks, weapons, grappling, restraint work - surely these must be an amalgam of techniques from various other styles? Well, no... because Systema doesn't have techniques as such, so how could it "borrow" them from somewhere else? It works through understanding key principles, which can be applied in any and every situation, confrontational or otherwise. No need to try and blend or force different arts together, when you can just study one thing and have it all!

This fact eventually clicked with me, and I discovered the best thing was to not try and pigeonhole Systema as this or that, or to compare it with the various arts I had studied before - but merely to accept it for what it was and just get on with the training. I suppose this was a version of the old "empty cup" expression.

To a certain extent, my approach has always been to try any new style with that mindset, to see it on its own terms and assess it from that perspective. Naturally, we all have our opinions formed by previous experiences, and we may also have emotional attachments to something we have invested so many years of training in. But I always had that curious streak. I was the one who asked the questions, who was always looking for something to fill the gaps

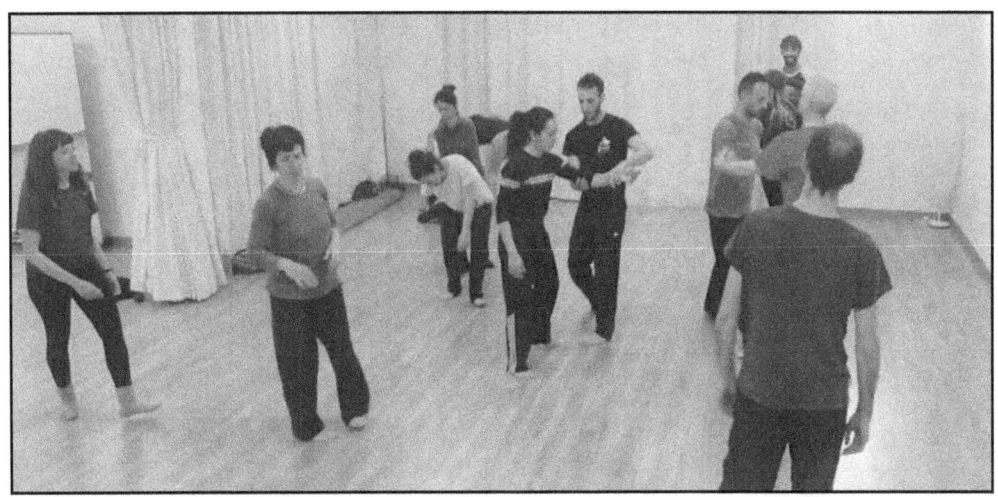

that I perceived in whatever I was studying (prime example, my former Chinese arts and groundwork.)

The perceived wisdom was, and still is to a large extent, study a boxing style for hands, BJJ or Judo for grappling, and Filipino arts for weapons. So there's three things I have to not only find the time to study, but then figure out how to integrate them all together. As I mentioned before, Systema is a one-stop shop. Its principle led approach means adapting what you know rather than learning a different set of techniques for each particular situation.

WHAT IS SYSTEMA?

This leads me to the notion of Systema being an *operating system* rather than a martial art. In fact, I rarely use the term "martial art" to describe it these days, though it's hard to find an alternative that people can relate to.

Now, as you've probably been training in Systema, or at least have some familiarity with it, this may well all be strikingly obvious - but it is highly relevant in terms of the contents of this book, which is advice for a Systema Instructor, because this is how most conversations go:

"Hey, I'm starting up a new Systema class on a Thursday, you should come."

"Great! What is it?"

"Well, it's a martial art."

"Oh, so standing in rows punching the air, no thanks."

"No, we don't do that, there's no set moves and it's good for self defence."

"Ah, you mean Krav Maga?"

"No, it's not that either. See we do all this breathing stuff."

"Gotcha! Like yoga, then?"

"Not really. I mean, there's no set moves."

"If there's no set moves, how do you know what to do?"

"Well, we work off of these principles. For

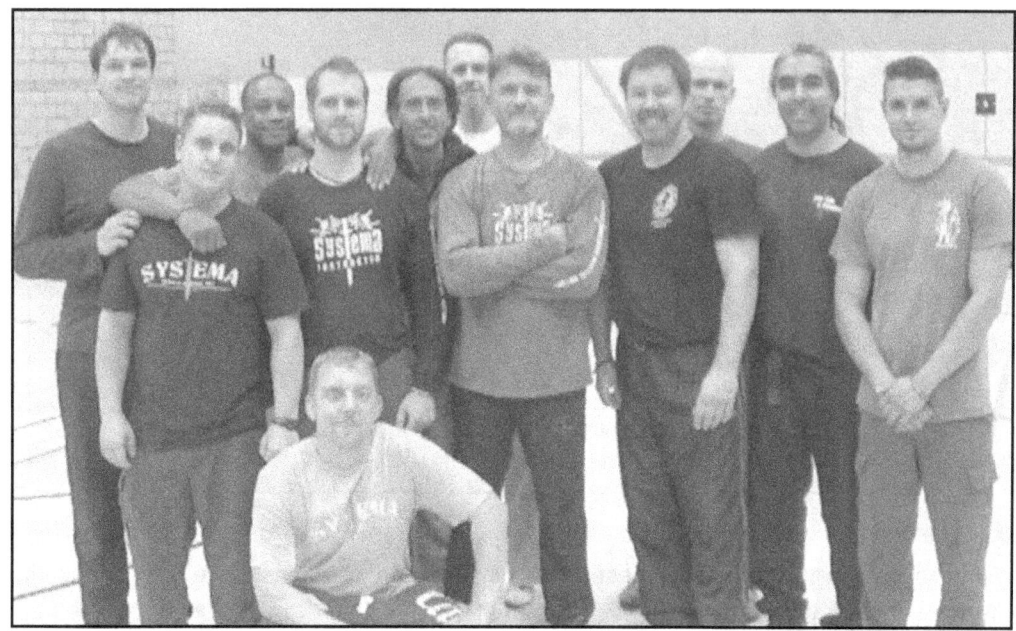

example -"

"Do I get a snazzy uniform?"

"Well, no, but -"

"Are there gradings?"

"Well, no."

"So how do I know how good I am?"

"Listen, forget the bit about martial arts, think of it as a kind of operating system. Oh, we hit each other, too. I mean really hit other."

"What? Hit? Er right, thanks, but I'm busy on a Thursday."

And so it goes. Naturally, as Systema spreads, which it has done largely to the efforts of Mikhail Ryabko and Vladimir Vasiliev, then hopefully that understanding of what it is will grow as well. But, at the end of the day, the mainstream will always try to reduce anything down to basic, digestible chunks that can be easily categorised, that fit neatly into a box. And inside the box is not where we want to be!

Alongside that, comes the challenge of lack of a formal syllabus. Given free reign to teach whatever you like, then what do you teach? I hope to answer this question, and many others, over the coming pages. I've been teaching martial arts full time since the early 1990s, and feel I have a few observations and ideas to bring to the table.

Of course, some of these ideas are universal - teaching is teaching. It is about communication, whether you teach physics, playing the trombone or boxing. Understanding your subject, presenting it in clear ways, challenging your students in a constructive way, maintaining your own levels of skill, these are issues to be considered across the board.

Alongside that, there are some things

that are universal when teaching martial arts - movement, generating power, mindset, and so on. Most importantly, of course, is that we are teaching things that are effective and fit for purpose. This calls for understanding context - a method for working against a kneeling samurai is rather specific to a certain time and place. There may be things we can take from that method, but what is the best approach to learn them?

In that respect, as a martial arts instructor, we should always be looking for ways to make our students better, faster. There's no place here for "secret" moves, for holding back information, for dragging out the training. I recently heard from a friend who re-visited his old traditional school from years back. Students were still doing the same basic footwork drill he'd been doing back then. The same material for years and years, with a promise of "one day we'll show you how to use it." No thanks.

By the same token, we have to recognise the abilities and deficiencies in students and teach them accordingly. So an older person's first session is not likely to involve diving over tables, for example. Maybe crawling under them is a better start point? To that end I'll also be talking about drills and how to develop and adapt them. Systema is marvellous in that respect, you have *carte blanche* to tweak drills, adjust them on the fly, even to make your own ones up! A person at a workshop once said to me, "you're making this drill up as you go along!". My reply was "Yes, that's what I was taught to do."

Alongside that, I'll be including advice on structuring a class, how to organise your school, running or hosting workshops, keeping an eye on your own development and also managing occasional difficulties that may pop up along the way. I'll also add in some class notes from past sessions to give you some ideas, and look at how you can develop into more advanced work.

Teaching Systema has, for me, been a rewarding, frustrating, joyful, exasperating, scary, challenging, creative, expressive, humbling and occasionally poignant experience. It has taken me to several countries I would never have visited, and forged close friendships both locally and round the world. It has been a method of true and honest communication that cuts across nationality, culture, class, occupation, age and creed; something that simultaneously allows us to share our common human experience and to each express our own, unique individuality. I wouldn't change a moment of it.

CHAPTER TWO
FIRST STEPS

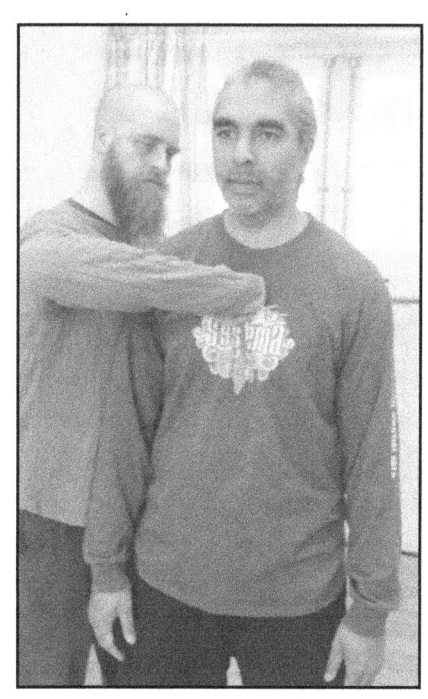

So you want to be a Systema instructor? The first question to answer, is *why?* Let's consider some possible answers.

THERE'S NO LOCAL SYSTEMA CLUB

This is quite a common one, particularly in the early days of Systema. Many of today's established schools started up with a few friends getting together and working from videos, with occasional visits to the main teachers. Often, but not always, there will be one or two people who take the lead, even if it's just in booking the hall and deciding what drills to do. This is a nice way to start, as you begin by working with friends, so there is less pressure to be "perfect." Everyone learns and grows together.

SWITCHING AN EXISTING SCHOOL

This was my own experience. When I came to Systema, I was already running a school alongside my colleague Dave Nicholson. Between us, we had clubs in the north and south of the UK, training in our synthesis of styles, based largely on Chinese martial arts. We began integrating more and more Systema in, until it became obvious that we should just switch over completely!

On the plus side, you will already have a club structure and student body in place. On the minus side, not all your students may be happy with the change, so be prepared for people to leave.

SOMEONE ASKED ME TO TEACH

Perhaps friends, family or colleagues are concerned about personal safety, and have asked you to teach them some self defence, or perhaps fitness, or mobility. Again, this gives you a ready made base of people that you already know to start with.

I WANT TO EARN MONEY

This is fine, there is nothing wrong with this, as long as you have realistic expectations. Just bear in mind that many of the people who make serious money in martial arts do so through pyramid-style schemes, through expensive franchise set ups, through charging for gradings, for taking a hefty percentage of earnings from people teaching for them, and/or from taking membership money from all students.

None of these are inherently bad, but they can lead to what, for me, is an overly commercial approach to teaching. It is interesting how you find that this tends not to work within the Systema framework. I have found that rip-off or ego-driven instructors tend to either stay away, or come and go very quickly in the Systema world.

Having said that, deriving income from something you enjoy doing is a great thing, and why shouldn't you? I've had a few experiences in martial arts, and many more in music (my other day job), where people say something like "hey, it's an art, you should teach for free!"

To paraphrase the reply of an elderly

Chinese Sifu that was once told this: "And will you feed my family?"

I've also found that giving things away for free doesn't work. I had a friend who was teaching free Taiji classes in a busy London park some years back. He was constantly disappointed by the very low turnout, even though he was a good teacher. Once he started charging, numbers picked up! By all means help out people who need it, but teach for free and not many will value it.

We all live and operate in a system that revolves around money, that's just a practical reality. You will likely incur expenses when teaching - venue hire, petrol costs, equipment costs, advertising. Not to mention the time that you put in to organisation and doing your own training. It is perfectly reasonable to be compensated for those at the appropriate level. But you must temper that with realism - you may think that Systema is the best thing ever, and that people will come flocking to your class. Be prepared for that not to happen - you may have nights were one, two, or even no-one turns up, it happens!

Of course, the pandemic over the last couple of years has wreaked havoc on all sorts of clubs and activities. So be prepared to be adaptable and take the rough with the smooth.

Always be up-front about fees, be reasonable and realistic and you won't go far wrong.

I THINK I CAN HELP PEOPLE

Mikhail once said something that always stuck with me. "People come to us as instructors because they need help."

It is true of all of us, though we don't always realise it, or understand exactly what sort of help we need. I would guess that people come into martial arts primarily because of issues around self defence. That may be down to bullying, to fear of crime, or for professional reasons. Alongside this, people want to get fitter, stronger, move better, meet new people, and so on. None of these motivations are exclusive.

An astute instructor learns to recognise what people are actually asking for when they come training, it's one of the first questions to ask a new student. But issues can often run deeper, or sometimes will not reveal themselves straight away. So a big

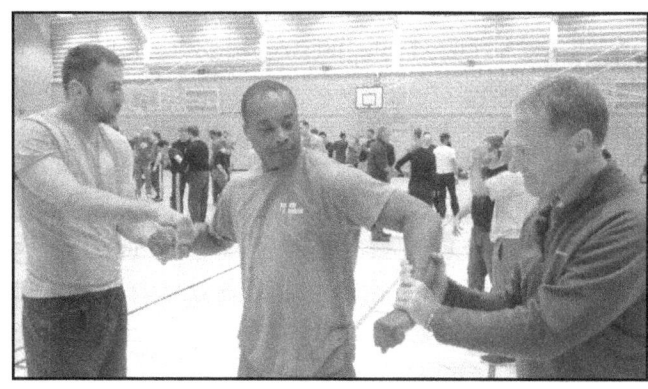

part of teaching is recognising how and where you can help people, in a variety of ways.

We should also be aware of issues that are beyond our ability to address, and be ready to advise and point a person towards the appropriate expert. As a simple example, a person may come into class who has very tense shoulders. If that is just down to stress, I can show them some exercises, breathing and movement that will help. However, if the tension is down to a medical issue or injury, I would advice that they also seek advice from a medical professional. Now, it may well be that I can offer supplementary exercises to help with the condition, but it is beyond my skill set to assess bursitis or a torn ligament, or so on. In short, stay in your lane.

I once saw a person insist on giving a back walk to a person with severe lumbar problems, the outcome was not good. This highlighted not only a failure of judgment on behalf of the instructor, but also the desire to help out "no matter what." Often this becomes about the person offering help rather than the person needing it. It can get a bit "look at me, I can help you!" Just be aware of that and temper any offers of assistance with tact and empathy.

I WANT TO HELP SPREAD SYSTEMA

Although it has expanded hugely in the last 20 years - I believe there are now something like 250 schools worldwide in the Ryabko/Vasiliev group - Systema is still relatively small in martial art terms. So there is still room for growth, though organic growth is better, in my opinion, than that driven artificially by hype and over-marketing. Over the past few years I've seen a few styles come and go that have relied on heavy promotion, flash marketing, expensive franchise buy-ins and eye-watering costs for instructor training. Typically, they make a lot of noise for a while, then disappear within a year or two.

I'm not saying we shouldn't promote ourselves, but I think we should do so via solid information and "sensible" marketing. The best way to do that is to simply present the benefits of training in Systema. We can point to the numerous health benefits, the effectiveness of application, particularly for professionals, the improvements it brings to fitness, mobility, etc, not to mention the stress management aspects. The challenge is in getting these benefits across, something we shall return to later on.

It's not uncommon for people coming into something new to be somewhat "evangelical" about it. That is fine and we all do it to some extent. Just be aware of keeping things honest, realistic and, above all, don't be a Systema bore! Also bear in mind that the people you are preaching to may well have considerable experience of their own. Don't put other methods down, instead stress how Systema can enhance other arts and activities, not just replace them.

I'M TAKING OVER A GROUP

Sometimes the instructor of an existing class has to leave - they might be moving out of the area, or so on. Rather than have the class fold, it may be that you wish to take it over. Again, the advantage is you have a ready-made base to work with.

I WANT TO IMPROVE MYSELF

I think most teachers in anything agree that the best way to learn more about a subject is to teach it. I don't hold with that old expression "those who can't, teach." It's nonsense, when you think of musicians, art teachers, boxing coaches, language tutors, etc, etc.

Teaching something like Systema does two things. First, you have to have a clear understanding in your own mind to be able to explain something. Second, teaching puts you under pressure and on the spot. People in class will ask all sorts of things. You may have to think of an answer quick, or consider something in a different light. Most importantly, it's okay to say "I don't know." Nor are you expected to be absolutely perfect at every aspect of Systema. *Who is?* Well, okay, maybe there's one or two, though I doubt even they would agree!

Students will generally understand the level of their Instructor, and cut them slack accordingly - especially if you are up-front and honest. This leads me on to our final reason, one I feel is very important and often misunderstood in the martial arts world.

I WANT TO BE KNOWN AS AN INSTRUCTOR

In many martial arts, being an Instructor, Sifu or Sensei, is seen as a rank - akin to being a black belt, or similar. It is a sign of experience, ability and status. This is not always the case, of course, we know that in less authentic schools, rank can be purchased, or awarded by people who you then award back! Rank may also be awarded to recognise commitment, or service to the school.

My personal opinion is that I don't think of *Systema instructor* as a rank - it's only a job description. You are simply the person who runs the group and supervises the training, that's it. You are not anyone's "master", no-one has to bow to you or call you a certain title. You're just the person who organises the sessions.

That means you may have only 18 months Systema training under your belt, or you may have 18 years. You may be a combat veteran skilled in several disciplines, you may be an office clerk who just enjoys Systema. Either way, if you are running the group, you are an instructor. This confuses some mainstream martial artists who view an instructor as some sort of pseudo-mystical figure - and the better they are, the more unapproachable they become, you have to earn the right to even be noticed by them!

An instant thing I noticed when first training with Mikhail and Vladimir, was the complete absence of that outlook. They talk to everyone, touch hands with everyone, train and teach everyone equally. Because that is an instructor's job, that is what they do! For me, this was a huge contrast to previous experiences, where a "master" would not even teach but have his seniors run the class, while he sat in the corner.

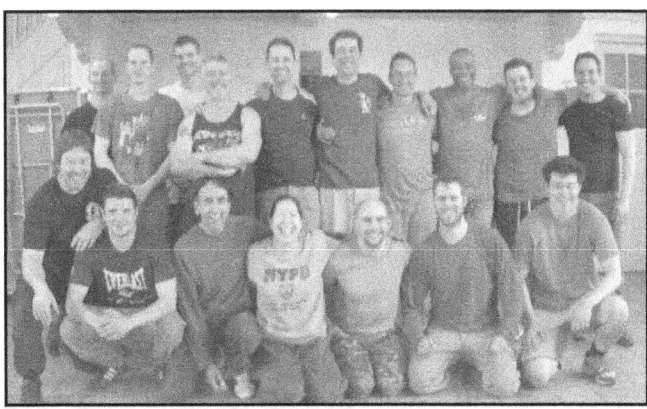

Those same seniors would Master's carry bag, even walk ten paces behind him when out and about. It was unheard of to get physical contact with the Master, especially at workshops. They would only ever demo - when they rarely did - on their own senior students. You see, there could be no risk of "loss of face."

The danger of this approach, something that I've seen first-hand, is that the Master becomes somewhat detached from reality. Not only in terms of only always working with compliant students, but also in terms of ego. One time I witnessed an irate Master phoning a local company to make a complaint and shouting at them "But I am Sifu X." Outside of the school, no-one cares!

Another aspect of this is where people come into Systema thinking they can become an Instructor purely as a thing to add onto their CV, to their list of ranks and achievements. They have little or no interest in the art, it's really just another stripe to add onto the belt. Again, without fail, I've found they very quickly fade away. Teaching for ego is a sure-fire route to failure, it is certainly not something to be encouraged, quite the opposite, in fact.

So is the role of the Systema instructor more like that of a coach? Maybe. We are back to our categories again, and it depends very much on how and why you are teaching and what you feel comfortable with. Again, just be honest about your capabilities, you don't have to be great at something in order to guide other people through it - at least in some cases. I will talk more about this later on.

These, then, are a few motivations for becoming an instructor, and, of course, they may well overlap or change as time goes on. The vital thing is that you have a genuine interest in Systema and in sharing it, and are open and honest in your dealings with people. Having talked about the *why*, let's next look at the *how*?

CHAPTER THREE
SETTING UP A CLASS

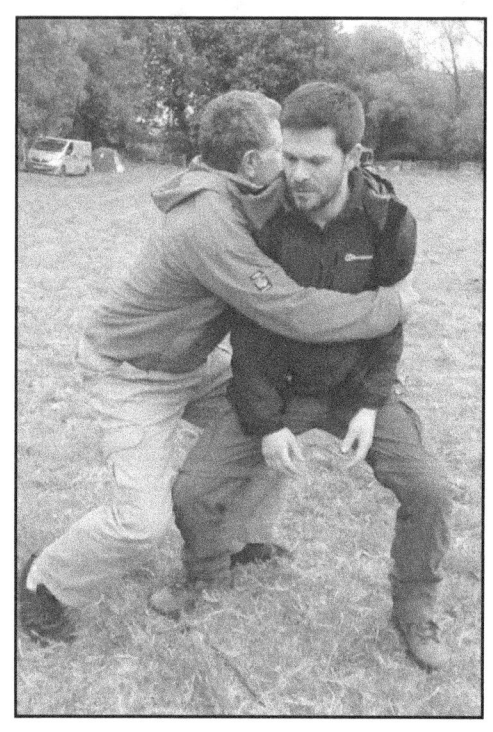

Establishing our reasons for teaching gets us started and, to some extent, will determine the next step - how and where we teach. I write from the perspective of being in the UK, of course there will be some variations in different parts of the world. Generally speaking, though, classes work pretty much the same wherever you are - you sort out a venue, organise a time, and, hopefully, people turn up! Let's start by looking potential venues.

SPORTS HALL OR GYM

A local leisure centre will typically have a gym, swimming pool and sports hall, with perhaps some smaller rooms available too. Dedicated gyms may have a training space or separate rooms for different activities.

Pros - good facilities (parking, changing rooms, etc), usually have mats available, good footfall, there's often a notice board or FB page to advertise on, usually in a central location that people are aware of, people can see the class going on and may be curious.

Cons - can be expensive, other activities may be going on in the same space, can be noisy (we used to train in a gym where the weight class below was accompanied by a pumping techno soundtrack), lack of privacy (an issue if you are doing knife work or pressure testing), busy places so maybe difficult getting a time slot, you need to be finished on the dot (often the next group are waiting to come in.)

DANCE / FITNESS / MARTIAL ARTS STUDIO

These usually have one or two sizeable rooms for hire.

Pros - nice sprung floor, mirrors, bars for stretching, good facilities, networking with instructors of other styles.

Cons - the time slot issue again, people may not like weapons training, there may be an "atmosphere" between different style instructors.

LOCAL HALL

This might be a church, a village hall or a community centre. These are generally funded by charities or local groups and act as central hubs for community events and projects.

Pros: reasonable hire fees, good local networking.

Cons: tend to be very busy, can involve quite a lot of red tape, basic facilities, hirer may be wary of some aspects of training.

OUTDOORS

There are fitness groups that operate entirely in local parks (though they have been prohibited in some areas). I also know of Systema groups that have trained in public parks (in one case police were called!).

Our Saturday group often trained at the rear of a public field in Tempsford. The area was a historic site, and was quite private. The fact that it was the site of a Viking battle

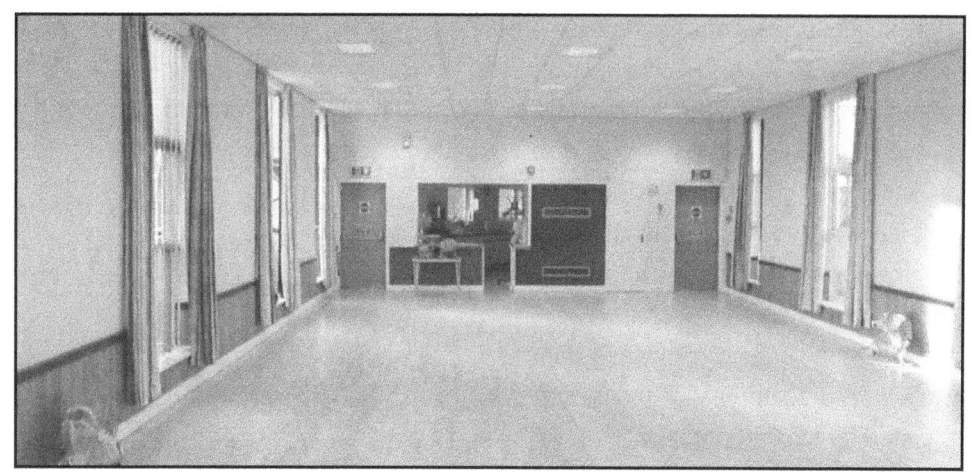

in the 7th century added a certain ambience! Of course, all our training camps are run outdoors.

Pros: Systema always feels better outside! Plenty of space, potential good obstacles for working round or climbing, good for training in different environments, cheap or free to use, no time pressures.

Cons: privacy issues, safety concerns, weather considerations, is the area easily accessible, no facilities, little or no footfall, dog walkers and joggers!

HOME
You may have a suitable training space at home, depending on your circumstances. Just first check that anyone you share the house with is happy with you inviting people round to train!

Pros: no travelling, all your equipment is to hand, no time pressures, control of the training space, low cost.

Cons: space / interference with family life, inviting people you may not know into your home, neighbours / landlord may object, no footfall.

WORKPLACE
This may be your own workplace, or you may be asked in to teach at a premises.

Pros: ready made group of people in place.

Cons: lack of space, having to move desks, etc, have to fit in around work hours.

I've run classes in each of these venues. For many years I ran a class at the main sports centre in Cambridge. We had use of a very large room (which I also used for workshops, including visits from Mikhail and Vladimir.) There were mats, changing rooms, showers, etc. You could also put posters up on notice boards, and got mentioned on the centre's website.

However, people had to pay not only to use the attached car park, but also a £1 entry fee to get into the centre. In effect, this almost doubled the cost of the class for people, or at least those who were driving.

Most of my teaching over the past ten years or so, has been in local halls. Each village in my area has its own hall and in Bedford, a large town, there are around five or six community centres. The issue with these is being able to get a time slot. What with yoga, dance classes, weddings and so on, you might find it difficult to get a space. However, I will say that post-pandemic, it has been easier - I guess a lot of activities have, unfortunately, gone by the wayside.

I mentioned training outdoors, something we will cover in more detail in the chapter on workshops, as there are some specific issues to address. I also currently teach from home, with a designated outdoor (covered) area that will accommodate half a dozen people. In some ways I prefer this, it is far less formal and there are no time pressures, in fact I see it almost as a return to the "old school" teaching of the past, it feels more personal.

First step then, is to check around your area for any of the above. The internet is usually the start point - though check with people you know, too, some of them may be attending pilates classes or similar at suitable venues.

Next step is to get in touch with the person responsible for hire. Send a simple e-mail asking what times are available, or what your preferred times are. I tend to say it is for a "fitness and self defence class." You don't need to get into the intricacies of Systema, keep things general. You might want to add a link to your website or social media page. If you do, be sure to check through it, as per the advice on promotion in a later chapter.

Don't forget to ask what the hire fees are. Locally, these can range from £10 per hour (local hall) to £30 plus VAT (local gym.) So check before you commit!

Once the hirer responds, make arrangements to visit the venue. Never hire a place unseen! Now, most places will be okay but there are some things you need to check:

Condition
Is the place in suitable condition? I've been in some places that could do with re-decorating, but that hardly affects the training. If there's holes in the floor though...

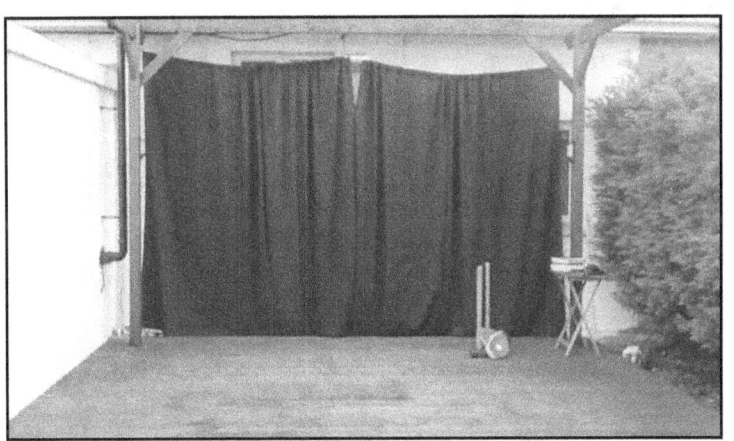

Accessibility
Is the place reasonably easy to find? Shouldn't be an issue with GPS, etc these days, But I still get people going to the wrong hall at my Bedford class!

Parking
Self explanatory. No-one wants to park three streets away and carry kit, or have to pay extra to park.

Area
Are you happy to leave your car there, that's usually a good indicator. Also, how busy and noisy is the venue? I used one place that over-looked a busy shopping area, meaning constant noise and traffic fumes in the summer.

Privacy
Are you happy with people watching what you are doing, or will this prove a distraction? This is most often the case in larger venues such as sports centres, but you may have other groups using a village hall at the same time. Do they have loud music going? Are people walking through your space to use the facilities?

Access
How do you get into the place? I am lucky at the moment in that all the halls I use have given me a key, so I can get in and out by myself. At other venues, I've had to wait for caretakers to open up, or similar.

One time in London, I advertised a new Taiji class. On the first night I had a dozen new students turn up. The caretaker was twenty minutes late in coming to unlock, and he moaned about it even then. As you can imagine, few returned the next week.

Training issues
Are the hirers happy for you to be doing what you are doing? I was once refused hire of a church hall for Taiji on religious grounds. Fair enough, it's their venue. You might also want to consider the use of weapons, particularly in the UK where the sight of even a butter knife can cause palpitations. How much you tell the hirer is up to you, but maybe don't rock up with replica guns on the first sessions - at least let the locals get used to you first!

I usually find that the hirer wants to meet me,

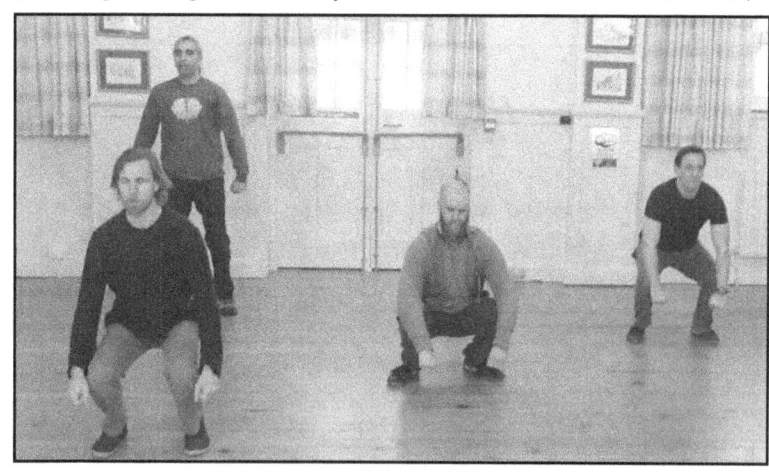

in person, which is understandable. I treat this almost like a job interview - the person is checking that you are an okay type to use their facilities. So turn up on time, be friendly, again, no need to go into huge specifics about what you do, keep it light and general. You may be asked for public liability insurance (I have been for most sports centre type venues), you may be asked for proof of qualification for teaching (in 40 years, only once!) so be prepared for that.

Remember to check about access, also make sure they give you a phone number to call in case of any problems. Some hirers who give you a key may ask for a deposit (this has been the case with local community centres) so you might want to take your cheque book too (do people still use cheque books?)

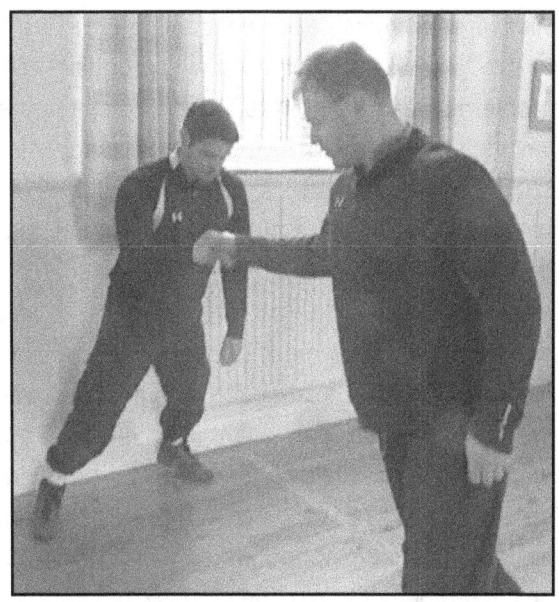

PAPERWORK

I mentioned certificates and insurance above, so a quick word about those. If you have been qualified by Systema HQ, you will receive a teaching certificate. You will also be included in the School Directory on the main site, and will have any enquiries for your area referred to you. Of course, you also have direct access to and support from HQ, and the wider Systema community in general.

As far as insurance goes, although I've never had need to use it - and have never heard of any other instructor using it - most venues will ask that you have Public Liability insurance (in the UK, at least.) You can get this by joining a martial arts group (though check their requirements. Years back, one group I was going to join stipulated rubber training knives, and to only work on mats.) Another option is to go direct to companies who insure fitness instructors, sports people, etc. This is usually cheaper. Currently (2022) I pay around £70 per annum for PLI.

You should also be thinking about first aid. Be conversant with at least the basics of recovery position, etc. It is quite easy to get formal training in first aid, or at the very least have a qualified First Aider in attendance. I always have a simple first aid kit at class, and maybe something more substantial if we are working with weapons.

Also run a survey of any new training area before you begin to check any potential problem areas. Indoors, these might include sharp corners, loose carpets, and so on. Outdoors, check for things like broken glass, holes in the ground (rabbit burrows often trap the unwary!), water hazards, and so on.

Having some element of danger does not mean you have to abandon training, but be sure that every participant is aware of the potential hazard. In fact, you could even construct drills based around first aid issues - for example, how would you carry an injured person out of the woods?

Also, think about how people are paying you. Cash - do you have change? By card - do you have a portable card reader? Be sure to have any forms or fliers on hand to give out as required.

PROMOTION

Alright - we have the time, we have the place, now we need some students to fill it! Promotion, for me, is the aspect of teaching that has seen the most changes since I started. Back in the old days, you put small ads in the local papers and put posters up in all the local shops. We also used to put on a martial arts demo, either at a local fete, or we'd to hire a hall and sell tickets to our own (these were usually very successful.)

I'd also approach the local press for articles, or get a reporter to come down for a free class - both newspapers and radio. That would sometimes lead to exposure in the wider media. In London I was once called in to Capital Radio, to "teach Taiji on the radio." Yes, I know... Still, it was good publicity.

Just a word of warning when dealing with the media. Aside from the trip to Capital, I've also been interviewed by magazines (such as *Maxim* and *Men's Fitness*) and had slots on various local radio shows. I can only advise that you be prepared! You may get a good reporter / presenter. You may also get someone who thinks you're a bit of a nutjob, but they have three minutes of air time, or two inches of column space to fill.

I remember getting a very good two page spread in the local Peterborough newspaper. The pair who came out asked sensible questions, and took some good pictures. In contrast, the *Maxim* interview on self defence advice, conducted over the phone, was reduced down to "Rob Poyton says if anyone attacks you, hit them with a brick." I'm not sure I even mentioned the word "brick" let alone gave that advice.

I also had a poor experience on a local Cambridge radio station, It was a breakfast show, meaning having to be up at silly o'clock (hey, I'm a musician, we're not morning people.) I'd organised a workshop on knife awareness at a local school. This was a session on awareness, avoidance, basic first aid, discouraging the carrying of knives and so on. In other words, a sensible approach for a particular age group. The presenter's opening comment was, "So, someone comes at you with a knife, you go HIIIIYAAH! and kick it out of their hand, right?"

To be honest, it threw me a bit, and I mumbled, "well, no." Actually, what I should have said is "I'm sorry, I thought I was coming on for a sensible debate about a very serious topic" and hung up. But there you go, you always think of the right thing to say after.

All I'm saying is, be aware, the media may not take you as seriously as you take yourself. It was for similar reasons I turned down an appearance on a Mel and Sue TV show a couple of years back. They basically wanted to ridicule musicians who played in tribute bands as being fantasists who thought they were actually Robert Plant, or whoever (no-one I met in any tribute band ever does, by the way.) The lure of mainstream exposure is often the bait on the hook of making some inane presenter look funny or clever at your expense.

But I digress! So, back to the modern age... Local newspapers and press seem to have largely disappeared, though that may be different in your area, and worth checking. I find these days there are very few places who will put up posters. Your local library perhaps or, most frequently, fast food shops! You might also check local notice boards. Don't be tempted to fly-post, you'll only get fined.

Another thing we tried was to have hundreds of small leaflets printed, then drop them door to door and hand them out at the local station to commuters coming home. I've also seen them firmly tucked under windscreen wipers in supermarket car parks. Not an effective method. Door to door or handing out, we never got more than a one percent take up, and delivering so many leaflets is extremely boring and time consuming!

Social media is the big thing now, though

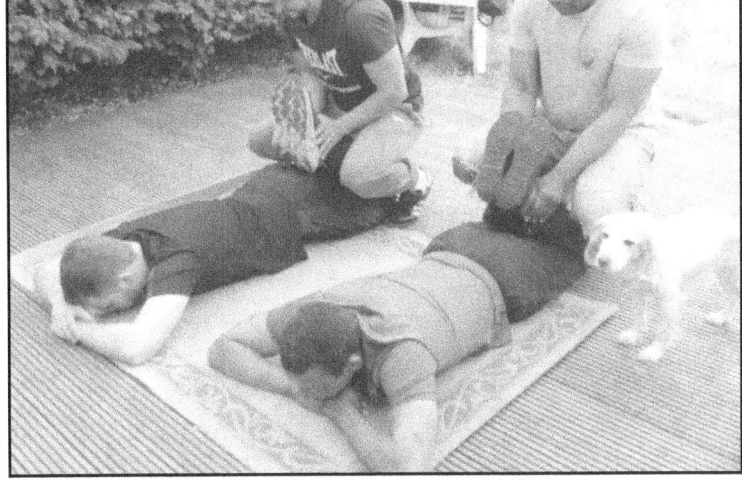

which particular platform is best needs to be considered. Where are your audience? Are they on Facebook, or Instagram, or Tik Tok, for example? See if there are local community pages on FB, these are usually a better bet than martial art pages. Just be aware of group rules when posting and don't think you have to make a post every day, that is usually counter productive.

I know you can pay for ads on Facebook. I've never heard of that being successful, but you might like to give it a try. You can also try posting on appropriate forums, Reddit groups, etc, though be prepared for negative responses - I'll talk a little more about that later.

DESIGN

Whichever advertising method you choose, you need to have appropriate media. So let's look at some tips for advert design, starting with flyers and posters

Posters and flyers
Think heading, solution, image and contact info. For example, if you are working from a self defence angle, the heading might be along the lines of
ARE YOU CONCERNED FOR YOUR PERSONAL SAFETY?
　The solution is
THEN TRY OUR SELF DEFENCE CLASSES!

The accompanying design should be appropriate and encourage interest. It should be a plain , clear image, perhaps of someone who looks like your target audience doing a movement. Avoid anything extreme. You might accompany the image with bullet points:

* BEGINNERS WELCOME
* EASY TO LEARN
* SIMPLE, PRACTICAL METHODS

Don't be tempted to go into deep explanations. I've seen posters that include a chunk of hard to read text giving the history of the art in details. It's off-putting. Bullet points are fine. Finally, give your contact info - a website and/or a phone number. I usually add *office hours only* under the phone

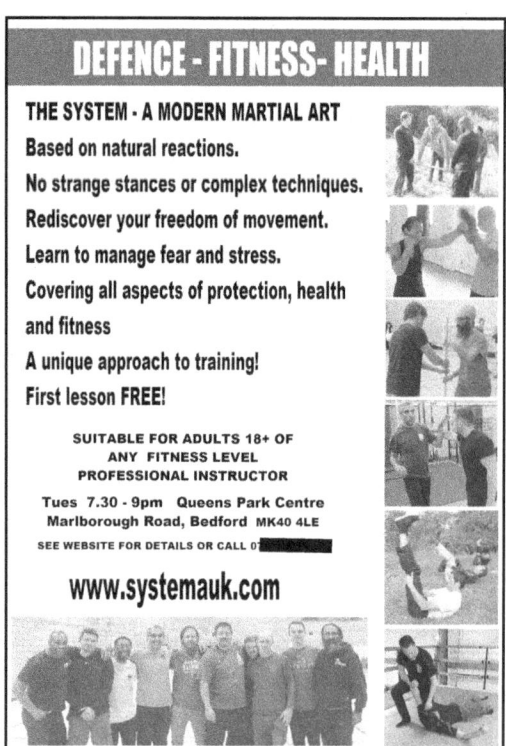

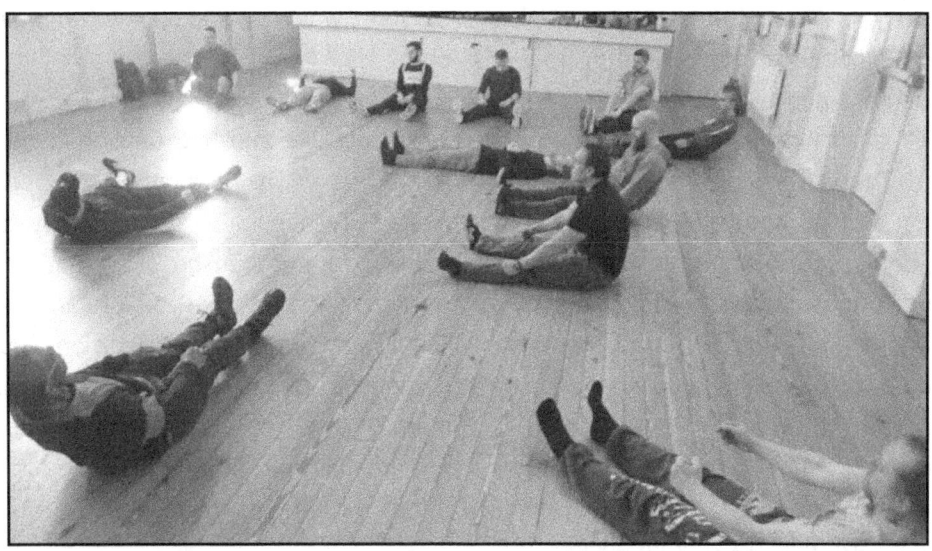

number, you'd be surprised how many people call at 10.30 at night. Make sure that you have your website up and ready. There's nothing more off-putting than going to a link that says *PAGE DOESN'T EXIST*.

Once you have all the ingredients, you need to put them altogether. Traditional headline colours are red or yellow in a clear, bold font. Avoid anything that looks like handwriting and especially avoid Comic Sans! I usually use a font like Impact or similar. Your bullet points and info should likewise be in a clear, san serif font.

Consider how large your poster or flyer is, where it will be displayed and how it will look from six feet away. Leave space at the edges for drawing pins, no point having a phone number that is covered up! You can print your own posters at home, or if you need bulk numbers, there are plenty of high street digital printers available.

SOCIAL MEDIA

If I have a good poster, I'll usually use that for my FB / Instagram, etc posts too. You have the added advantage of being able to add a direct link in to the post as well. Posts with images or videos always get more attention than just plain text, so even if you don't have a poster, see if you can add a suitable picture to a post.

Video

If a picture is worth a thousand words, a moving picture must be worth a million. Approach your video as though it was a moving poster, with the same design principles in mind. Keep it short and simple, show people training and having a good time. Quick cuts, no explanation, clear bullet points and contact info.

Unless you are a great presenter or have acting experience, don't stand in front of the camera and talk. Let the training sell itself, make it look fun, effective and not too tough. This is a difficult one, as if you show all soft training people think it's too easy and not worth doing. But show students taking punches and kicks and going through extreme exercises, and people will think it's too difficult! It largely depends on what your target audience is. Pitch the video accordingly. If you are aiming at door staff, then set up a few short door-work drills, for example. Keep your editing tight.

You can use background music for a video, what you use is a matter of choice. Personally, I avoid heavy metal and go for something with a bit of a beat and a simple riff. Listen to TV shows to get some ideas then, if you have the resources, make your own. There are also copyright free clips available (or you can commission me for a reasonable fee!). You can use someone else's music, or a famous tune, but you may run into copyright issues and, if posting on Youtube, you won't be able to monetise the clip.

With phones, Go-pros, etc it is easy to get footage and photos these days, and there are many editing apps and programs available. It's worth investing a little time in learning basic editing, you will likely be using it a lot. I also always have a camcorder on-hand at class, useful for getting those little clips, and for other reasons, which I will explain a few chapters on.

There a still some "old fashioned" forums around, as well as FB groups and places like Reddit, Twitter, etc. Posting on Systema-specific forums can be okay, but posting anywhere else can get you into arguments! Then you need to make a decision - do you respond to negative comments, or ignore them? It is very easy to get dragged into long arguments that quickly degenerate into name calling and mudslinging - and for what?

I remember Vladimir talking about this once, as even he gets negative comments on-line. His take was to shrug and say, "What's the point? You can't convince anyone over the internet, and they never turn

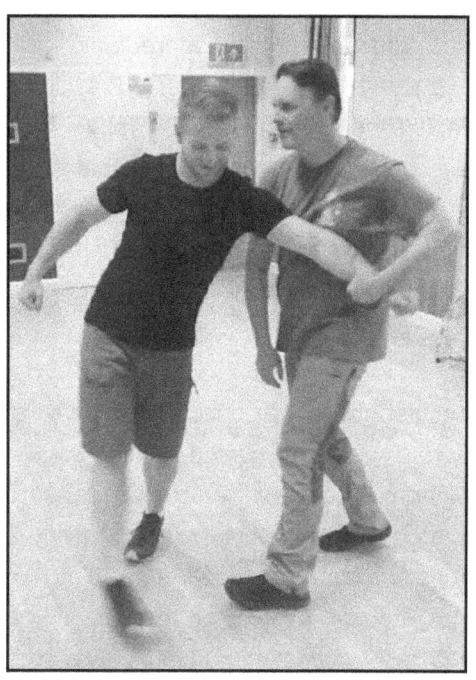

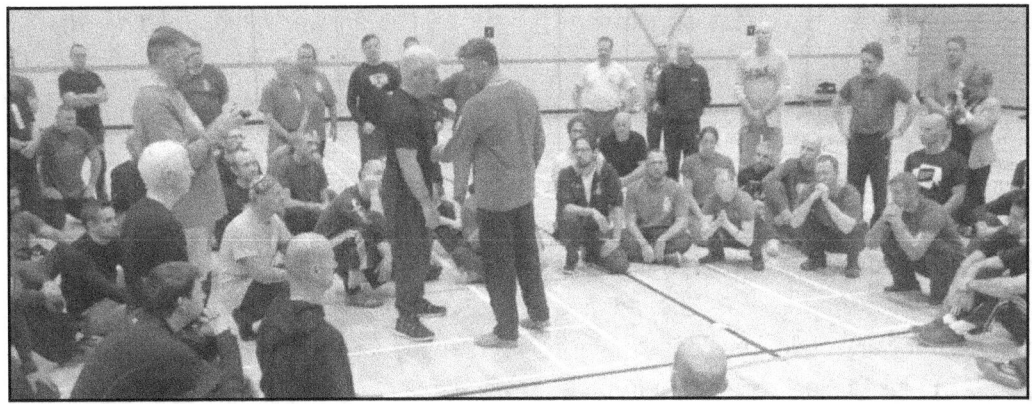

up to test it."

When the internet was still quite new, and I was in my "evangelical" phase, I used to respond a lot to comments. I remember a particular exchange, it might have been on the Bullshido forum, that went along these lines.

"Systema is crap. Ryabko is useless, I could knock him out."

"Great. He's coming into the UK soon, the venue is not far from you. You could come along."

"I'm not paying to do that crap!"

"I'm the organiser, you can come for free."

"But I won't be allowed to do anything!"

"You can do what you like. Only two conditions - you sign a waiver, and it's filmed."

"Yeah, but what rules would we be sparring under?"

"What?"

"I use British Kickboxing rules."

"Like I said, you can do what you like."

"Well, if you can't agree the rules, I'm not coming. Besides, I'd only embarrass your teacher in front of the class."

"Again, you can try what you like."

"Yeah, well, see, well...."

Of course, it was a no-show.

This was pretty typical. One guy even said he wouldn't turn up in case "Mikhail hypnotises me." You have to also remember, half the time you don't know who you are actually talking to. It might be an actual person, it might be a troll with an agenda. Even if it is an actual person, you don't know their abilities or mental state.

I was recently following some posts on a martial arts forum where a poster was making a lot points, he sounded like a real expert. Two weeks later, he put up a training clip of himself that was... interesting. My feeling is that he has some kind of issues, perhaps he needs some help rather than being castigated on-line.

So, it's up to you how much you get involved in this kind of thing - if nothing else, see it as way to practice your stress control, and never send your first response! If someone is making direct accusations against you, that is another thing.

A post on one martial arts forum claimed that Systema was a con, that instructors are all frauds. I posted to ask which particular aspects of my teaching and activities were fraudulent? The admins stepped in and told me not to "get personal." Like being accused of fraud is not personal! It was clear they were siding with that particular view and didn't want any mention of Systema on their forum.

Hopefully, once you have adverts out, you will start to get enquiries. What is the best way to handle these? Personally, I prefer e-mail or text these days, where I can add in links to my site, or cut and paste info. Some people like to chat though, but be prepared! When I first started teaching I would often be on the phone for 45 minutes plus, chatting about my art, answering questions about this and that, and so on. Quite often, the person wouldn't even turn up! These days I like to keep phone calls short and to the point. Give relevant information, keep any details about the training brief. I usually say, "the best way for me to answer your questions is in person, through the training."

Of course, some people may be nervous about attending, they may need some reassurance. Or it may be that they have some specific consideration they would like to chat about. That's all fine, do your best to answer without getting drawn into protracted conversation. I mentioned earlier about putting "office hours only" on your posters, etc. So if you get a call at 11pm, don't feel obliged to answer it, let them leave a message. Again, this is why I prefer e-mails!

Overall, by far the best method of student recruitment is word of mouth. This means that new people coming in have some idea of what to expect. They aren't coming in "cold" so to speak and, to an extent, they are "pre-screened." By that I mean, if one of my students brings someone , I know that person will be sensible. I've even had a student say to me "I wouldn't bring friend A, he's a bit of an idiot!"

PRESENTATION

Alongside the idea of advertising, comes the general issue of how you choose to present yourself. It can be useful to step away and take an outside view of your image. In the early UK days, a lot of new to Systema people were wearing ex-military camo gear.

From my perspective, this was for a few reasons. It's what we saw the main teachers wearing, so we thought "that's what people who do Systema wear." There was also an aspect of making those instructors feel comfortable when they came over to the UK to teach. Also, that kind of gear is hard-wearing and practical for training. There was also an element of who could get the most

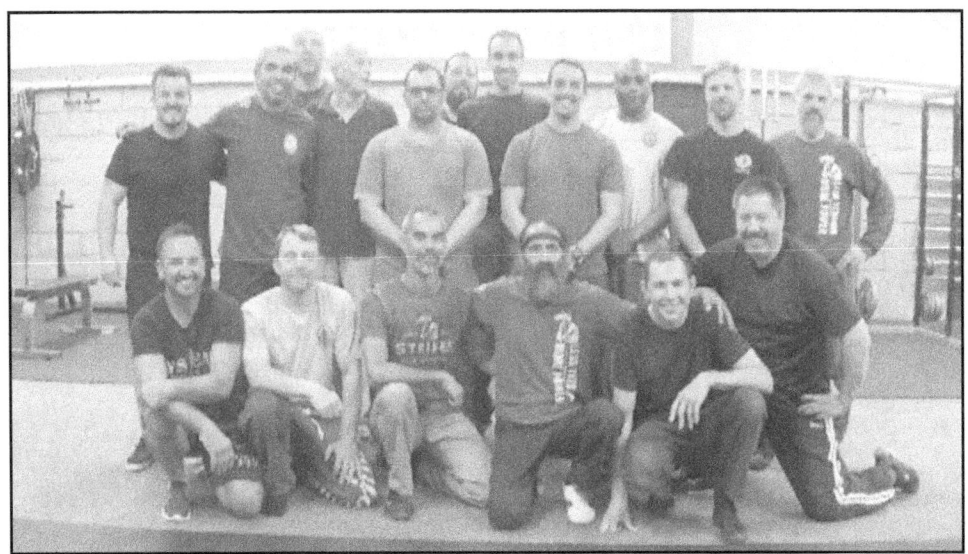

obscure or unusual camo pattern going on for a while! No-one was ever told what they had to wear, that's just the way it worked out

Matt Hill (former Para Captain) told me that when he came to the first big seminar with Mikhail and Vladimir at Cambridge, he walked into a room of camo-clad students and wondered if we were all some kind of Walts (military wannabes).

More concerning was a couple of lads telling me they were apprehensive at first coming training because of the military look - in their experience, it had associations with some UK racist groups. Thankfully, they came in anyway, but I sometimes wonder if others were put off.

These days, people wear whatever they like, from drill pants to track suits to jeans. If you are happy training in it, you can wear it. Of course, even then you can't win. A traditional martial arts teacher once castigated me for what my students wear. He was used to lines of people each in a crisp, white gi, I suppose, but each to their own. We should remember that for some, training is a form of ritual, complete with costume and "correct" procedure. For me, it's just a part of my regular life, I try to attach as little ritual to training as possible.

So, we have a venue, we have some students, next we need to think about the class itself.

CHAPTER FOUR
RUNNING A CLASS

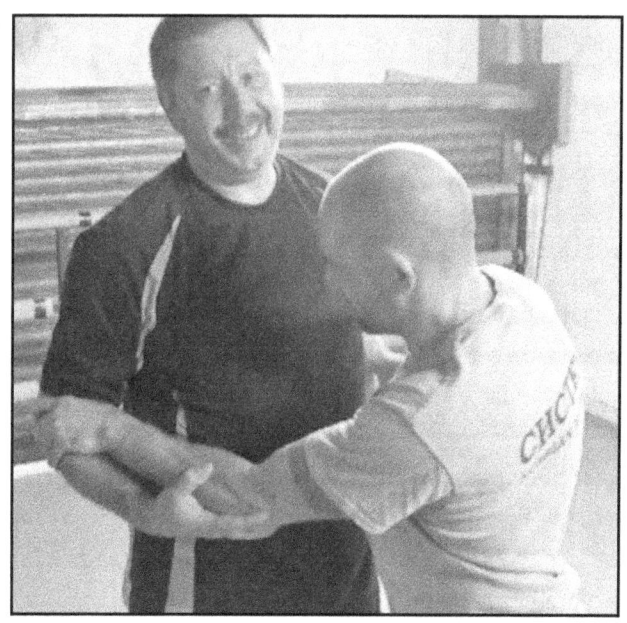

Before we get on to what we teach, let's first look at how we teach. You need to decide on your class format, what sort of atmosphere you want, the standards of behaviour expected, and so on. Anyone who teaches in any context will tell you the same thing - It is quite possible for one person behaving in a bad or inappropriate way to spoil the class experience for the whole group. Likewise, you need to carefully gauge the flow of information, and the intensity of training, as well as being aware of any potential "flash points" between students. But before all that, let's think about class length.

For a general Systema class, I like to teach for 90 to 120 minutes. I feel this gives a good time in which to warm up, run through a progression of drills and have some time for massage and questions at the end.

That will vary if the class is on a specific topic. For example, an exercise or breath-work only class will run for 45-60 minutes. For longer work, usually on a specific topic, I run workshops of between 3-6 hours, or occasionally a full weekend. These obviously give you scope to go into great detail into a particular area and/or to include a wider range of topics.

Finally, training camps or residential courses can run from 3-7 days. These will usually involve a team of instructors and allow for true immersion training. This is my favourite of all formats, but of course it involves considerable time and resources.

FORMALITY

Your class length will determine its structure, but let's first think about what type of class you want. Are you the sort of instructor who likes to stand at the front and have everyone follow along? Do you like things to be formal and quiet, or are you happy to have people chatting away as they train?

I tend towards the latter, preferring to keep things very informal. Everyone shakes hands as they come in and leave, everyone is on first name terms. I'm happy for people to chat as they train, in fact in some ways I encourage it. I say this because I find it helps people to stay relaxed, and also reinforces the idea of training our nervous system rather than learning rote technique. I want people to be able to react naturally in a real situation, not have to switch into some sort of pre-programmed mindset. Training "naturally" helps with this, it also helps students get to know each other.

Of course, you don't expect people to talk over you while you are explaining something. Also, the idea is that people talk *while* they are training. Sometimes, in challenging drills, people use talking as an excuse to stop and come out of the drill. Keep an eye on that, it can be contagious and, before you know it, the class has ground to a halt to listen to someone's joke or anecdote.

Don't be afraid to take control every now and then if required, or, as I usually do, get people to drop and do 20 push ups as "punishment."

You may have a different approach, and find that people respond to a more disciplined environment, that is all down to your personality. Even so, I feel that people learn Systema better in a more relaxed atmosphere. Then again, I am mostly teaching experienced people these days - they have developed an internal discipline. If you are teaching newcomers, or younger people, you made need to adjust accordingly. Speaking of which, I'd just like to mention here something about student motivation and the idea of goals and rewards.

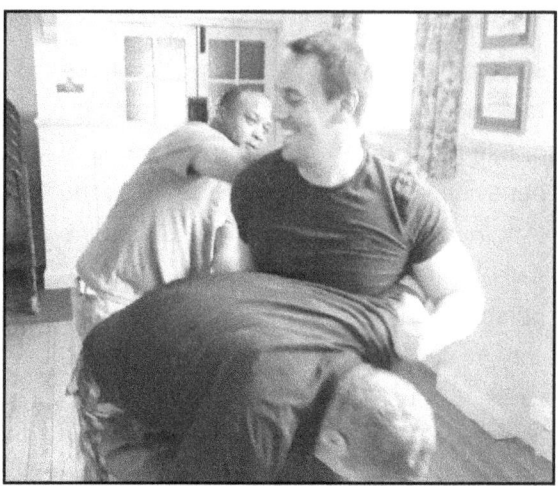

MOTIVATION

As we know, some arts use a grading structure to denote rank and reward effort. This can be thought of as an external reward - you receive both a physical item and a measure of status amongst your peers as part of the process.

An internal reward is more nebulous. It may be that you have set a goal yourself, say being able to hold a static push-up for five minutes, and have finally achieved it. No-one gives you a belt, they may not even notice, but you have the satisfaction of that achievement.

Or, think about the last time you did something purely for the enjoyment of the activity itself? For example, you may do some gardening, paint a picture, play a game, take a walk, or read a book. These may not produce something or provide a prize. Instead, we do them because we like to. They make us happy. This is another example of internal reward.

Researchers have discovered that offering external rewards for an already internally rewarding activity can actually make the activity less intrinsically rewarding. This phenomenon is known as the *over justification effect..*

"A person's intrinsic enjoyment of an activity provides sufficient justification for their behaviour," explains author Richard A. Griggs in his book *Psychology: A Concise Introduction.*

"With the addition of extrinsic reinforcement," Griggs writes, "the person may perceive the task as over justified and then attempt to understand their true motivation (extrinsic versus intrinsic) for engaging in the activity."

This distinction is now being recognised in the military. Research at West Point in the USA showed that even when factors such as race, religion, gender, socioeconomic background, and scholastic scores were considered, cadets with primarily internal motives were about 20% more likely to make it through training than the average. Cadets who did not have primarily internal motivations had worse than average chances of graduating. These cadets also had a 10% lower chance of sticking with a military career and a 20% lower chance of being promoted early.

This is part of a trend in education, too. Teachers today generally strive to develop learning environments that are intrinsically rewarding. Many traditional paradigms work from the approach that that most students find learning boring, so they must be extrinsically goaded into learning. In old school day terms, I remember this ranged from being awarded gold stars for good work to being caned for "infringements!"

In a book chapter called *Making Learning Fun,* authors Thomas Malone and Mark Leeper suggest that this does not need to be the case. They identify several different ways to create learning environments that are intrinsically rewarding.

Challenge: people are more motivated when they pursue goals with personal meaning and when attaining the goal is possible but not necessarily certain. These goals may also relate to their self-esteem when performance feedback is available.

Control: people want control over themselves and their environments and want to determine what they pursue.

Cooperation and competition: intrinsic motivation can be increased in situations where people gain satisfaction from helping others. It also applies to cases where they can compare their performance favourably to that of others.

Curiosity internal motivation is increased when something in the physical environment grabs the individual's attention (sensory curiosity). It also occurs when something about the activity stimulates the person to want to learn more (cognitive curiosity).

Recognition: people enjoy having their accomplishments recognized by others, which can increase internal motivation.

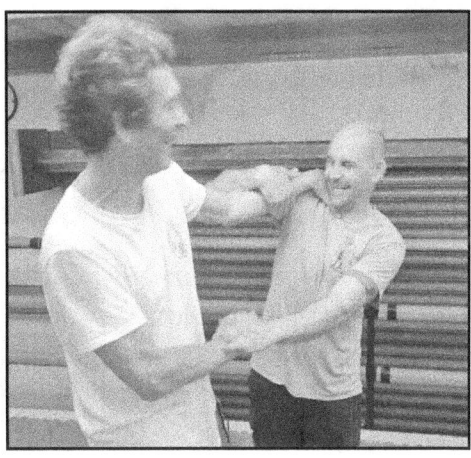

Bearing all this in mind, how do we motivate our students? The above give us many clues, which we will building into our drill creation and structures later on. For now, we can think about he we act towards students. Should we encourage them, praise everything they do, or never so much as crack a smile?

The answer, as usual, lies somewhere in-between the two. Praise where deserved, encouragement when required, criticism where necessary. I remember getting all three in one go when I first met Vladimir! He took me easily to the ground a few times, but then said, "Your balance is quite good." He followed that with a few handy tips.

Within a couple of minutes I was simultaneously pleased with myself, physically "destroyed" (in a nice way), and given advice on how to improve - all delivered with a smile. Interestingly, at that same event I saw Vladimir chastise someone for dangerous behaviour, but again all delivered in a calm, but certainly firm way. As my colleague Ed Phillips often states "sometimes the lion needs to roar."

Praise is best delivered in small doses. Too much, and it loses impact, never, and it is discouraging. If a student does something good in class, or shows an improvement, I'll always acknowledge it. A simple "nice", or a pat on the shoulder is enough. Incidentally, other students will also do the same, something that makes Systema classes so pleasant to train in. Your fellow students are genuinely pleased when you "get it."

Over-praise can often have a negative effect. I mentioned this once to a person who was being "too nice" to new people in class, or at workshops. The particular individual would work with them and, whatever the newcomer did, would tell them, "Wow" That's great! That's amazing, that was really, really good!"

It wasn't, the person was just doing the drill. I explained that it is good to encourage people, but if someone feels they are "amazing" in the first five minutes, why would they come back? They already learned everything! Also, you don't want to

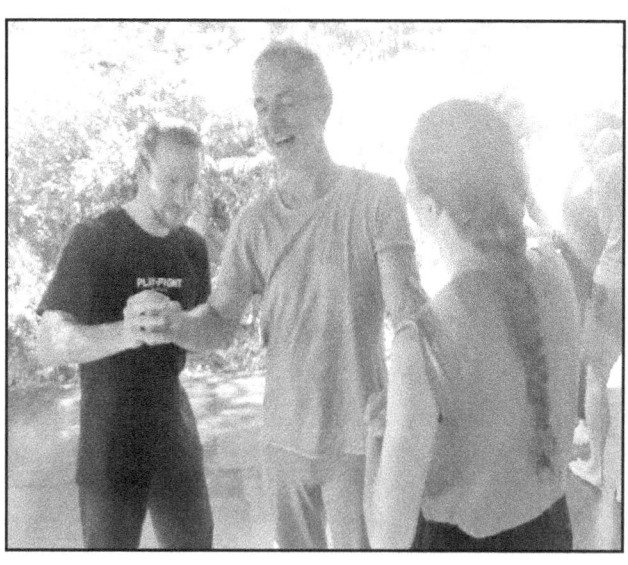

give people false confidence. Another aspect is that people might find it a little patronising to be spoken to like that, especially if they are more experienced in martial arts than the person telling them. Give praise, then, but temper it, don't let people become prideful, or feel that they constantly need to seek your approval.

On the other side of the coin, how should we approach criticism? One thing I learnt from my instructors is the approach of, "what you are doing is good, but have you thought about trying it this way?"

This is a much more constructive approach than saying, "no, that's crap, it won't work. Our way is best." And yes, I have heard that said, though not in a Systema class.

This is where the "professional mindset" aspect of Systema comes into play. When you talk to and train with high level professionals - from whatever field - you find they have a thirst for improvement. If you can show them a way to do something more efficiently, more effectively, they will jump at it. They understand you are not attacking their ego by making suggestions, you are helping them improve their skills or attributes. This is the way to present your work, by appealing to that internal motivation.

FEEDBACK

By the same token, an instructor should always be prepared to listen to students, too. Everyone has something to offer, everyone has experience in something. This especially struck me on my first training visit to Moscow, where Mikhail often let other people and instructors speak, particularly those with relevant skills in the topic we were training. This also helps move us away from the idea of a teacher as some kind of supreme being, all-knowing, all-wise, invincible. It is, sadly, an issue in martial arts, and breeds a very unhealthy atmosphere both for teacher and students.

Again, a Systema Instructor is a person there in order to create a suitable environment for people to learn in. If that means passing part of the class over to an expert, then by all means do so. Be aware of who you are teaching and don't try and show off, it rarely ends well.

I experienced both sides of this a few years back when a friend invited me to teach as part of his personal security day. This included work on dog handling, removing people from cars, close protection work and so on. I was running through some CP drills when the question of firearms came up. One of the students stepped forward and offered some tips. Now, I didn't know his exact history, though I knew if he was part of my friend's crew he would have a solid military background. His advice was on-point, practical and sound, I had no problem in "giving him the floor," I learnt a few things, too.

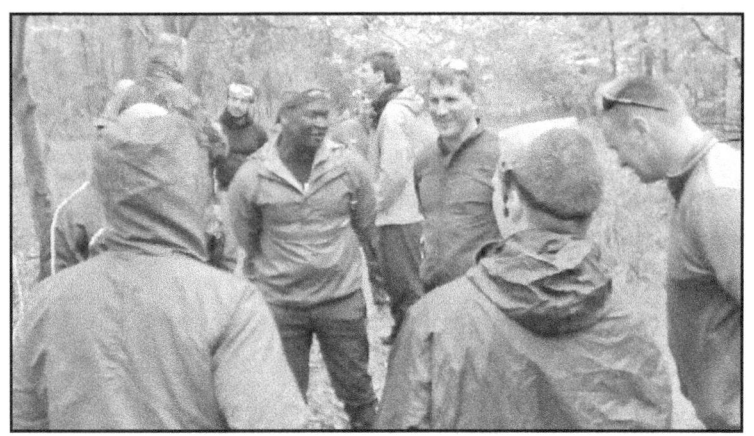

At the same event, another person tried to impress the assembled group with his "getting in an out of a car" skills. Quite unprompted, he began diving in one window, out the other, and so on, work that all of the group were quite familiar with. Of course, at one point he got stuck halfway and floundered, leading to someone remarking drily "Well that didn't pan out so well, did it?"

So, much like you would in any situation, social or professional, learn to read the room. Don't bluff, don't bullshit, and be sure to present your material without ego.

BANTER

I mentioned about people chatting while training (at least during some drills.) It reminded me of the time one of our lads took a grading at his Aikido club. He dealt very well with all his attackers, did everything required for the grade... but was failed. The reason given was that he was "smiling too much and this is a serious business!" In typical style, he laughed this off!

I also once garnered some criticism on-line about a knife workshop video clip, in which some students were laughing. I was told that and "there's no room for laughter in training!" I beg to differ, for reasons I have already stated. I'm not one for pulling "war faces" and shouting and screaming, fine as part of a scenario drill, perhaps, but not as a default setting. It's a popular approach in some styles, personally I find it all a bit "acty" - more Will Ferrel than real feral.

I've found that adults are perfectly capable of operating effectively without grimacing and pretending to be tigers or wolves - again, this harkens back to our concept of "professional mindset." Having said that, part of our training calls for heightening the emotions and triggering the nervous system, something covered in detail later on.

So I'm happy to have people talking and laughing in class, where appropriate. Humour is good, however, you have to be careful with banter. There are some professions where "banter" is part of the culture, where it seems acceptable, even expected, to put your colleagues down, to give people derogatory nickname, or to make comments based on certain features or characteristics.

I find this less productive in class and something you need to monitor. A person may come in with low confidence or self-esteem. Shouting "Oi, fatty!" across the room is not likely to help. Banter often slips over into bullying, which may be something a person has come to class to get away from. Again there is a place for it in some, and I stress *some*, drills but overall, I ask that everyone treat everyone else with courtesy and respect.

Naturally, as people get to know each other and become friends, humour can become more personal, but even then it should be tempered with an awareness of other students in class. It's exactly the same as reading the room that we mentioned earlier. Would you tell a filthy joke in polite company? Just apply the same standards in training.

There is a side issue from this too, which is talking in class about religion and / or politics. Both are potential inflammatory topics and I see little need to discuss either during regular training. I once had a guy coming to class who, as soon as he was in the hall, start talking about a particular religious group in derogatory terms. I'm not sure whether this was just the way he was, or if he had been sent to fish for new recruits for some organisation or other. Either way, it was inappropriate. After being told about it a few times, he eventually stopped coming altogether, so I suspect he may have been on a fishing trip. It does happen, and is something you need to be aware of.

CONSENT

Issues can arise if you have a mixed class, and again this is something you need to monitor. My classes tend to be mostly male, though some of our other groups are more mixed, and there are one or two women-only self defence sessions in operation, too.

As an instructor, it is your job to make everyone feel safe, supported and welcome into the group. A big part of that is the notion of consent - we train with consent. Make it

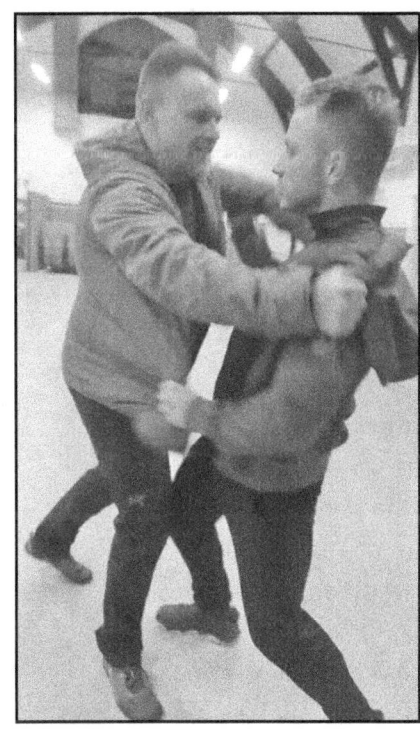

very clear to new students, and also remind the old ones from time to time, that we train with consent. The training might be soft, it might be challenging and intense, but it is always with consent. Everyone has the options to step out of a drill at any time *without judgement*.

This is very important. Encouragement is one thing, but being overly judgmental can backfire, something I once discovered, following an incident that still makes me feel ashamed.

I had not been teaching long, in fact I was still really just assisting at my teacher's kung-fu school. Two new guys came in, brothers. The start of the class involved holding a particular stance for around ten minutes, not as easy as it looks. One of the brothers started shaking and trembling after a minute or so, he was obviously struggling.

Now, these were both young, strong looking lads, so I made a jokey comment about "oh, you're not so strong then." I later found out that the brother I said that to was under-going treatment for leukaemia. Thankfully, I met the older brother a couple of years later, and had the opportunity to apologise to him. So, two lessons - don't judge a book by the cover, as they say,

you don't know what stresses, illness or traumas a person is carrying. And second, always encourage, don't deride.

As part of the consensual aspect of training, also make it clear to students that they should listen to their partners. If a person says "slow down," you slow down. If they say "speed up," you speed up. Don't dish out what you are not prepared to receive yourself.

In mixed classes, proximity issues can arise, with feelings of unease on both sides. I think this is something that women in general handle much better than men - but then, unfortunately, they have to. For example, I had one male student who, when training with a female partner, was obviously getting... excited. Short term solution, quickly have people switch partners. Long term solution, a chat and keep him away from female partners, though in that particular case he left the club soon after.

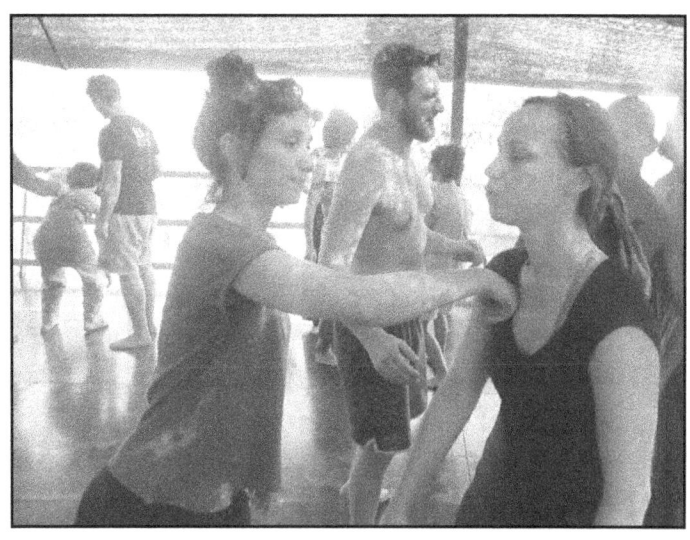

Likewise, don't treat your partner as though they are made of porcelain. Let them be your guide at to levels of contact, intensity, etc. Personally, I try put issues of gender or anything else aside and just think of the person in front of me as... a person. Each of us is different, we have different triggers, levels of tension, strengths and weaknesses. I've had huge muscle-bound guys in tears and pencil thin women take heavy shots. A big part of your job as an instructor is to assess and work with a person as an individual, not as a stereotype.

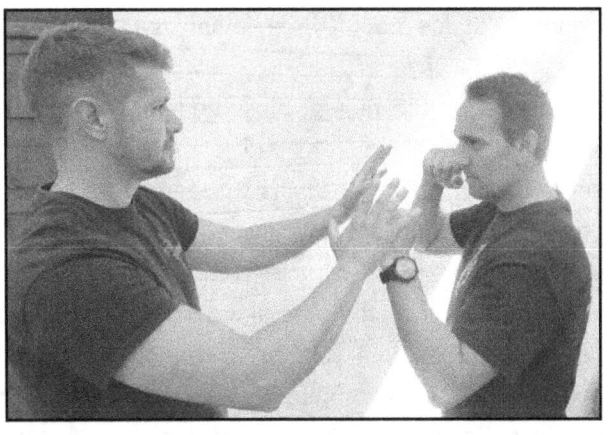

Always be mindful that people may have particular issues - injuries, for example, or perhaps cultural issues that need to be factored into the training. If in doubt, ask! I have trained with some Sikh people and always asked before doing so, if was okay to touch their beard or turban during a drill. All it calls for is a little sensitivity which, let's face it, is a prime Systema attribute.

All of these factors will combine to give your class its own atmosphere, added to, by your own and your students' personalities. There is nothing to say that every session has to be a certain way. You might want to have a "light" session, with more chat and fun drills, or you may be working in a more intense environment which calls for more focus and discipline.

We have run some air-soft sessions, for example, and there's no room there for jokingly waving a pistol about, even if it's "just" an airsoft. It's mostly common sense, Systema is just like life, sometimes you can ease off, sometimes you should push forward.

One thing that, in my experience, is unique to Systema is the Circle Up. At the end of the class, everyone sits in a circle, we go round one by one, and everyone gets the chance to comment or question. This helps reinforce the consensual aspect of training, as it gives everyone an equal voice and input into the session. I always add that people should talk without interruption from anyone else, this is their opportunity to speak.

At camps we carry out a longer version of this drill, following a format I got from Konstatin Komarov at one of the Canada camps. It's a powerful exercise that helps bring the whole group together, and gives people the opportunity to voice things in a supportive space that they may otherwise keep locked away.

Yet even in the regular class setting, I've heard everything from bad jokes to constructive criticism to new insights about a drill. Students have given advice based on their expertise, and shared both good news and bad, from the birth of a child to the tragic death of a partner. I cannot recommend highly enough that you include a Circle Up at the end of every session, it really is an amazing practice.

While talking about consent, we should also cover the issues of insurance and waivers. In fact, let's tie this in with how you welcome a new person to class.

First step is to make sure you are at the venue on time, or even a good ten minutes beforehand. This allows you time to deal with any access issues and also to be on hand when new people arrive. I'd advise you have a folder with you containing any flyers, forms, etc that you might need.

If your class is totally new, you can address the whole group. If you have one or two new people coming into an established class, you can take them to one side. Introduce yourself, thank them for coming, then give a quick run down of the class - how long it runs for, the rough structure, the idea of consent and so on.

I tend to put a lot of this info on a flyer that I hand to new people, along with fee structure, contact details, a little about my own background and so on. It's always good marketing to give people something to take away with them, it can act as a reminder!

I also ask people to fill in a form, including their name, address, DOB and contact e-mail / phone. It explains on the form that no details are stored electronically (data protection) and is used for my info only. There is also a space for people to note any injuries or issues they have, and a space for them to sign and date. They need to sign to acknowledge the waiver on the bottom of the form - I will put a waiver example in the Appendices.

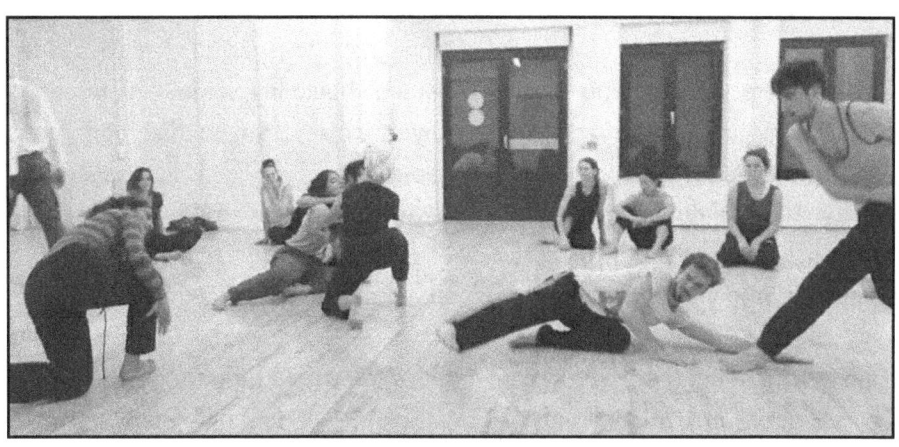

I collect personal details for two reasons - one, I like to know who I am training, and two, I add them to my mailing list (with consent.) They also have the option to join our WhatsApp group, an easy way to keep everyone in the loop about potential class changes, events and so on.

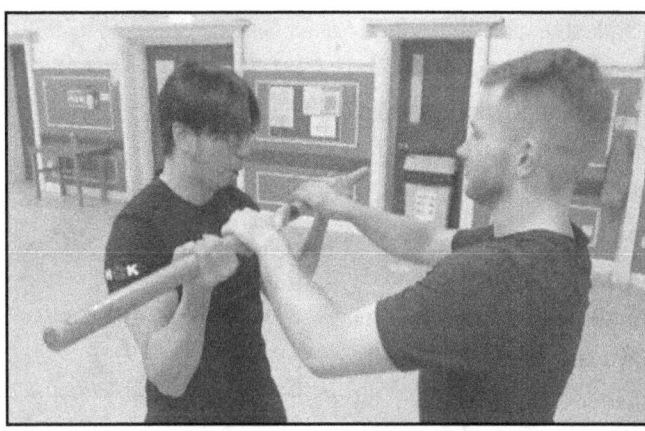

From there, ask if they have any questions, though keep answers brief. As with the phone call, taking part in the actual training is usually the best answer to any question. Be sure to double check for any injuries or issues - even then be cautious. I once had a guy come to regular training who had a pacemaker that he neglected to mention. That day we were doing heavy strikes to the chest, fortunately he was okay, and actually told me about it the end of the class!

Another question you might get is from a newcomer is, "Can I watch the class." Personally, I say no these days, for three reasons.

First, Systema can be deceptive. For example, slow push-ups look easy when someone else is doing them. You need to feel things first hand to appreciate them.

Second, Systema is not designed to be visually attractive or flashy. Often an experienced person is able to visually appreciate good or subtle movement. For those expecting flashy moves and spectacular techniques, though, the training can often look dull or even, ironically, "unrealistic." Remember, a person's view of "realism" may have more to do with action movies than actual experience. As Vladimir often says, "professionals view things with a different eye."

Third, people watching a class can have a negative effect on the students who are training. They may feel they need to "perform" somehow, or it might put them off their work, particularly if running more intense types of drill.

Admittedly, I will temper that according to the person. If it is someone who is clearly a little nervous, then I may make allowances. However, sometimes you get people who just want to watch "for a laugh." or similar. I remember, when I used to allow people to watch, at the Cambridge class, a young guy came in and sat there for the whole class. I think we were doing some joint locks and striking work. Anyway, he had a dismissive look on his face for most of the time. At the end, I went over to him, asked if he had any questions. His response was "oh, so you don't do any ground work, then!" and he walked out. Had he stayed a moment, I could have explained if he'd joined in the class he could have asked to do ground work, but there you go.

To be fair, mind, you can get the same attitude even when people join in. I've had people in to train for the first time and always make a point of asking during the session, if they have any questions or want to try things out. Once or twice I have heard of those people going away and saying "oh, I don't think that would have worked", or "why do it that way," or even, my favourite, "yeah I could have..." The time to raise these issues is during training, not later on.

FEES & MEMBERSHIP

Should you give a trial lesson? There's another question - first class free? I've tried free and pay for the first session, neither seems to make a difference to retention. It may be a marketing incentive to put on posters, but I've found that people will turn up if they are interested, regardless. How you structure your fees is up to you, here's some ideas.

Pay per class - students pay as they arrive or at the end of the session. Make sure you have some change on you. Or you can now get apps or small readers to take card / Paypal payments.

Pay per month - students pay on the first class of the month for the month ahead. An alternative (my preferred option) is to have people set up standing orders that pay direct into your bank account.

Pay per course - students pay up front for a block of classes or specific length of course.

Pay annually - quite rare, in my experience, though I did have one student who preferred to pay for six months at a time.

It is customary to offer different rates depending on how people pay. For example, your fee per class may be £12, a month may be £40. You may also charge different rates depending on whether people are younger, unemployed, services personnel and so on. You may also charge less if they are a club member.

It is quite common when joining a martial art school, to pay an annual membership fee on top of the class fees. This is something I personally no longer do, for various reasons, including admin and the fact that I prefer a more informal approach. If you wish to try it, then think about what benefits your members will get. These might include:

Discount on class and workshop fees
Priority booking for events
Access to extra training sessions / club events
A club T-shirt
A membership card or booklet
A regular newsletter
Student insurance
Gradings - not something I've seen in Systema classes so probably not relevant

Some schools, like gyms, run levels of membership, such as Gold, Silver, Bronze, each with its own price and rewards. I run a three tier system for my Youtube Member Channel, with benefits ranging from accessing all our instructional uploads through to live personal Zoom training sessions.

Whether you choose single or tiered membership, be sure to cost out your benefits. That might include cost per item for T-shirt printing, insurance costs and so on. If you are a member of an official martial arts group, they will probably offer student insurance at a price per head. Or, as with PLI, you can go direct to a company and purchase a block of student insurances.

Even if you offer student insurance, I would still advise getting people to sign the waiver as mentioned before. I'm not sure they have much strength in law, but they do at least show that you have given notice that training carries risk. Again, as long as you are professional in your approach you should have no problems.

One last thing to consider while we are talking about money - how much should you charge? It is impossible to give a figure as there are so many factors to consider. Do a little research and find out what others are charging in your area. Balance your costs with perceived value and price points. There is a school of thought that says if you charge more, people will value it more (similar to

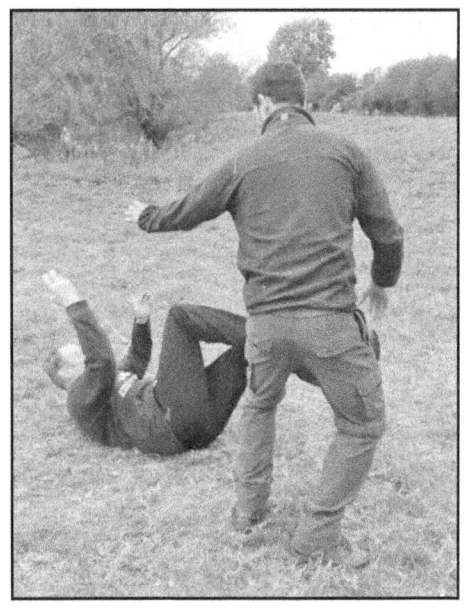

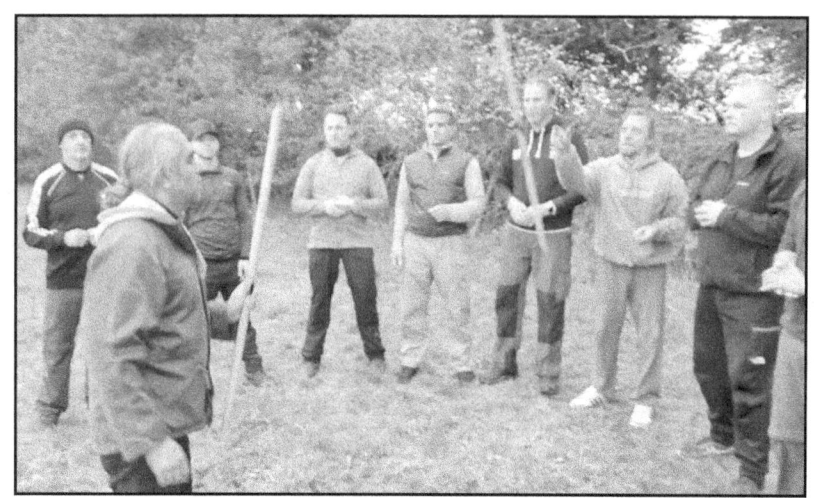

what we said about free classes not working.) However, there has to be a limit to that, which will depend on the area you are teaching in, the local economy and so on.   There is nothing wrong with offering discounts to students, unemployed, emergency service workers, etc. I've always said I'd rather have a good student fallen on hard times come for free than not come at all, so be flexible in your approach.

By the same token, be aware of people who may, try and take advantage - they "forget" to bring their money and will pay you next time, or similar. Now we all do that now and then, but I did have one person who tried it on regularly. Have a quiet word and remember, it is your class, you have the option to exclude people if necessary.

As I mentioned, my personal preference is for students to pay by monthly standing order. This means I know that my hire costs are covered for the month. It also demonstrates a measure of commitment from the student. I'm much more invested in students who turn up regularly than those I see three times a year (presuming they are local.) It should be obvious that progress in any endeavour only comes about through regular training. Of course, there may be good reasons for patchy attendance, but it does make things tough if you are trying to establish a new class.

You will probably find you get a core group who are there virtually every week, another group who come once a month, and then those students who drop in and out, even though they tell you how great the class is and how much they enjoy it. For this reason, it makes sense to have people on standing order. If you rely on pay as you go, you may find yourself struggling when the bills come in, particularly if you are using several venues.

You might also consider the option of one-to-one / private training. Again, check what local personal trainers and the like are charging and set your price accordingly. As with classes, you can offer the same payment structures for personal training. For regular sessions, I run for an hour. If a person has to travel a distance, or can only see me once in a while, I will run two or three hour sessions. Half a day is enough for anyone. More than that and people struggle to take in information.

I remember when I first started giving private lessons, having a guy book a full day of training with me. He wanted to learn "all the basics", so an early part of the day was on falls and rolls. After ninety minutes he'd said he'd had enough and left. I was in no way beasting him, he just found the training overwhelming. So now, unless I know people and/or they are experienced, I recommend just an hour session to start.

Some people think, particularly if they come from a background in certain other arts, that having one-to-one with the teacher will somehow give them access to "better" information. This is probably a hang-over of the Chinese tradition of having what were known as "indoor students," literally, students who would be invited to the masters house for "secret" training. These are the students who would go on to become official disciples in the style. That doesn't exist in Systema. No-one is special and we are all special!

Of course, one-to-one you get personalised training, the focus is all on you. However, you also miss out on the benefits of training with a group. The same information goes to the group as it does to the individual. So by all means, use one-to-one to tighten up on specifics, or if no regular group is available, but don't see it as a short cut to learning all the secrets. There aren't any!

EQUIPMENT

Do you need equipment to start up a class? In general, no, at least there is no specific kit you need, as opposed to training in Kendo, or similar. In fact, no-one even needs an outfit, though you should ensure that people are wearing appropriate clothing. One lad used to turn up in steel toe cap boots - no thanks.

Typically, we do not train on mats either - though if you have some available, you can

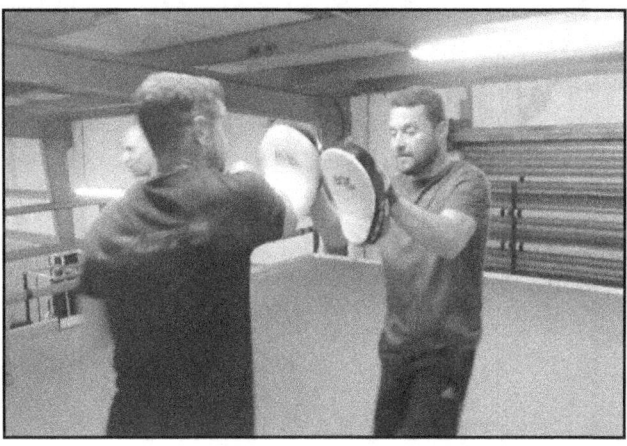

use them, particularly for beginners or more challenging falling work.

However, as you go through, you will find there are numerous bits of kits that will cone in useful These include:

Sticks - a sturdy stick around 4' in length is the single most useful training tool you can have. Short sticks are also useful.

Focus pads - useful for speed training, developing power in strikes, awareness, breath-work and a few other things beside. Standard boxing type pads are fine, maybe a thicker elbow pad and/or kick shield.

Knives - most styles use rubber knives for training. The only time we use these are for full speed drills, and not always then. For close in work they are useless. Use strong plastic knives, even better, use blunt metal knives. Butter knives are fine, or similar light trainers. Real knives, blunted, are another option. We occasionally work with live blades too, but only with experienced people. What type of knife you use is dictated by the nature of the drill. To truly learn fear control and precision, you need a metal blade. For faster work, use plastic (and even then wear eye protection)

Protective gear - eye defenders, padded helmets, shin guards, etc. Again, all may be useful depending on the drill. We sometimes use bag gloves for sparring, or more padded gloves if we working, say, the short stick against a hand wielding a knife.

Any padding has pros and cons - people feel confident to work faster, but the feedback is less realistic. I recently bought a body shield that will take full power body shots, at least to the front. Nice for the punchee, but the feedback for the puncher is horrible! Still, they are useful for positioning and speed.

Also be aware that padding doesn't always

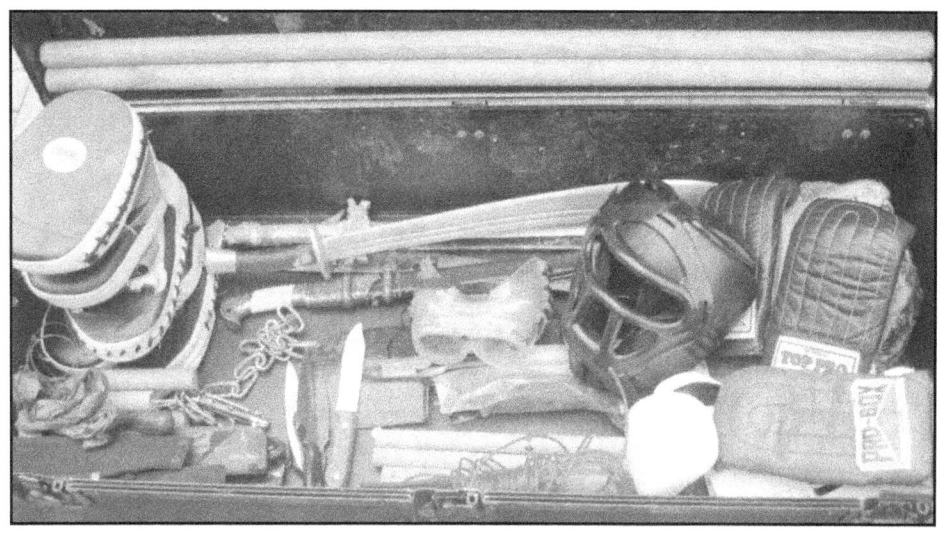

protect. The first time we tried a power slap to a padded helmet, the recipient was stunned by the impact. Remember, as well, that wearing large boxing gloves, for example, not only affects your fist formation but also changes the range a little - plus you can use them as a shield, which you cant rely on in real life.

Other weapons - be sure that they conform to local laws. Replica guns for training disarms, airsoft for handling and shooting, swords, flails, anything and everything can be used.

Improvised weapons - chairs, clothing, various every day items - can all be incorporated into training. These may be already at the venue, or are things that students can bring with them.

Should the instructor provide all the equipment for training? At one time, I tried to. So every class, I'd be hauling round a bundle of sticks, a bag of knives, a holdall full of pads,etc. I soon got fed up with that! So now I advise all new students to get those items themselves. Again, with an eye to the law, they can bring pads, weapons, sticks, etc to class with them.

A serious student should have all these things in any case. Also, when people say "can we do some work with the short stick?" and everyone has one, the answer is - *yes!*

Just one other consideration when it comes to training weapons - be sure to check everything before it is used. People are normally sensible but I have had someone get out a live blade with the intention to use it in a training blade drill. Take nothing for granted!

ONLINE CLASSES

The recent pandemic saw many of us having to shut down classes and stop teaching face to face for a while. An offshoot of this was the rise in online classes. Fortunately, technology is currently at a point where most of us can run classes via the internet with decent picture and sound.

While there are obvious limits to teaching this way, I found that Zoom classes, at least, kept the group in teach with other. It has also meant being able to keep in contact and train under my own teachers, as well as chat to other people around the world. So let's look at some of the pros and cons of direct online sessions.

Pros
No hire cost for premises (assuming you have space at home)
No travel for students, so, potentially, a global audience
Class times are easily adjusted
Sessions can be recorded

Cons
You might not have space at home and there may be interruptions
You need a decent internet connection

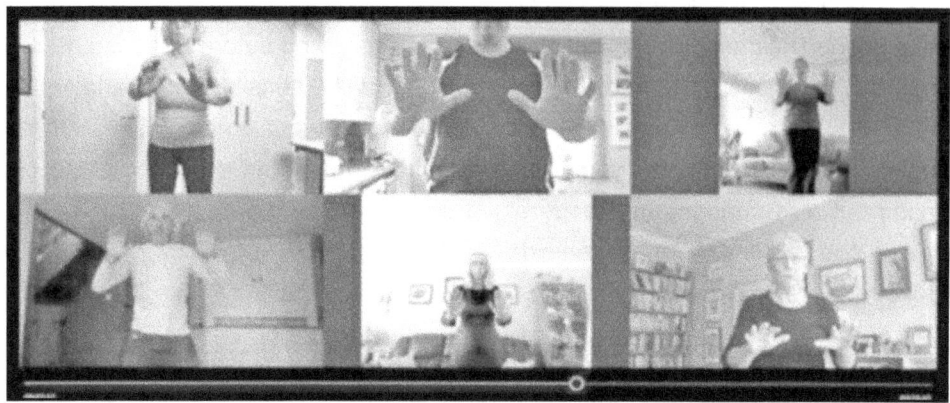

All teaching is visual, no tactile component. It may be difficult for people to follow your movements

You have no control over the training environment as a whole

Students may be alone and have no partner to train with

I personally found that online sessions work best for exercise type classes. It is easy enough to have people do various types of exercise, be they movement or breathing based. It is also possible to run through attribute training - things such as balance, ground movement, stick work and so on.

If students have partners, it may be possible to show some movements or techniques. You may have someone helping you, in order to demonstrate. The teacher can then watch the students and advise on corrections. However, there is obviously no "hands on" correction possible.

Another possibility with this format is to give talk and lectures, something I have been asked to do a few times. These were mostly based around stress management type work, so the only physical component were some breathing exercises. In these cases, online is an ideal platform.

Even now that lockdown is over, I still run a couple of Zoom sessions a week. They are mostly exercise / breath-work based, with the occasionally "normal" class. If you wish to try the same thing, work through the following checklist.

Equipment - a standard laptop set up is fine if you are sitting and chatting. If you are further back from the camera, showing movements, you may want to look at getting an external camera and microphone set up - these can be bought quite cheaply and will generally do the job.

Lighting - think about where you will be filming - how is the light? Your indoor lights may be enough, if not you can buy basic light set ups quite cheaply. Go for LED, a simple white light with a filter screen across it is best.

Background - what can people see behind you? A messy room? People walking past? I always prefer to film against a neutral background, so I either work with my back to the large hedge that runs alongside my training area (if the weather is fine!), Or use a curtain suspended from the ceiling if filming indoors.

Sound - do you have a quiet space or will there be background noise? As I write, we just have a new puppy join the household. He can be very barky at times, which can be challenging when running a "quiet meditation" session, so bear your surroundings in mind!

It might also be worth getting your students to "mute." I found that, quite often, people's phones are ringing, or someone would comes into their room for a chat, or the doorbell rings, all things that can be off-putting to instructor and other students!

If you wish to record the session, be sure to let everyone know and give them the option to switch their camera off. Not everyone likes being filmed.

Another option for on-line training is Youtube. You can produce uploads that are accessible only to people with the direct link. This has most of the same pros and cons as working via Zoom or similar, though of course the training is not "live." However, I've been running a member channel for a few months now, and find that it is working well. Members from around the world can send in a question which I can answer, on film, within a day or so. Sometimes I do this alone, other times I take that question into a regular class and film the answer there.

In short, then, online training is great for some types of work, not so good for others. It can put you in touch with a world-wide audience, you might even think about using a Zoom group in order to build up and launch a live class in your area.

KIDS CLASSES

One other subject to discuss before we move on, is setting up specific or specialised classes. One is example would be teaching children classes. This is not an area I have experience in - the youngest group I ever taught was when I was called in to run a self defence course for a local Sixth Form college, with students around the 17-18 age mark.

Other than that, I've never had any interest in running kids classes, though we have often had people bring their children with them to train, which is nice. Bearing that in mind, I will offer a few general ideas for child-specific classes, but first make a recommendation to someone who is having great success in teaching Systema to kids.

Tommy Floyd in Florida now has a download out that gives a lot of great tips

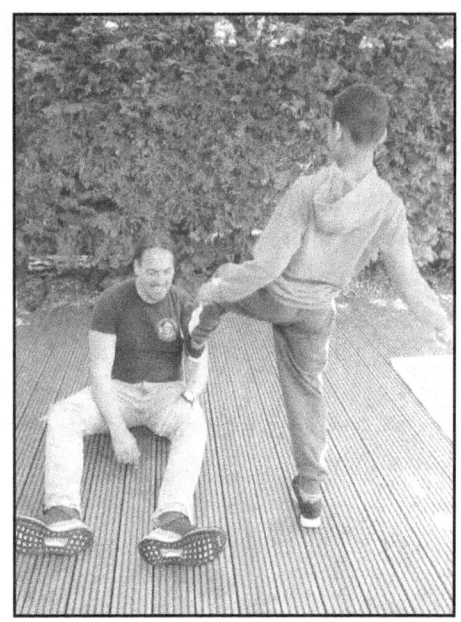

and advice for structuring and running a child class. I will place the link to Tommy in the Resources section at the end of the book. I will also post a link there to an excellent article by Konstantin Komarov, part of which I reference below.

Now, with its "playful" aspect, Systema is an ideal martial art for young people. The emphasis on free movement, spontaneity and creativity is much more healthy for kids than having them stand in rows repeating movements - in my opinion. This play mode should then be a major foundation for the class.

First, think about age ranges. We might divide these as follows:

Up to 7 years old – training in small groups, using games that require a lot of movement.

7-13 years old – think active, mobile, developmental games, plus specialised exercises, and a lot of wrestling.

14-16 years old – introduce the basics of Systema, using specialised exercises, wrestling, and strikes. At this age you can already put the children in some adult classes, but until then it's better to keep the groups separated.

16+ year-olds can usually participate in adult classes.

Syllabus aside, another consideration when teaching children are any local regulations or laws pertaining to child protection. In the UK, it is usual to have what is known as a DBS check , as well as having a child protection policy in place - so be sure to take this into account. It may also be worth seeing if you can get one of the parents in to assist, as you may find children need more management than adults.

SENIOR CLASSES

At the other end of the age spectrum, you might look at teaching older or elderly people. My oldest student to date has been a gentleman in his eighties. Systema is one of the few arts that can do this, in fact many of its aspects can help people in later life.

Obviously this type of class will largely focus on mobility and health training, but you may well find there is an interest in the application side too, particularly if students have previous martial arts background. If that is the case, I have generally found that older people fit in fine with a regular class.

But if you wanted specifically to target seniors with little or no martial art interest or experience, it is entirely possible to do so. And, of course, you needn't put any age restriction on the class either, my health classes run from teenagers to retirees. The key is to present exercises that can be carried out by people of any condition. Take a simple balance drill, for example, just lifting the foot and holding the position for a while. Some people may like to use a chair or the wall for support. Others may only be able to lift the foot a few inches off the ground. There may be those who can lift the knee up to waist height. In this way, everyone can be doing the exercise but at their own level of comfort and ability.

My health classes run for 45-60 minutes and always start and end with breathing. In-between we do a lot of stick exercises, some stretching, joint rotation, balance and so on. Recently I have run two workshops for older people on learning how to fall safely. We started on thick mats on the ground, helping people to first of all relax on the ground. As it happened, one of the participants tripped over three weeks later, and tucked in her shoulder and rolled out to the side - job done!

I do find that many of my seniors are more wary of contact type drills - such as gentle pushing on the shoulder, massage and the lie. However they do enjoy group exercises such as stick gauntlets! There are a full range of suggestions for this type of work in my book *Systema for Seniors*, but it should be quite easy to extrapolate drills from your regular classes and tweak them where necessary.

DIFFERENTLY- ABLED

Something of a catch-all title for students who may have physical disabilities or neuro-diversity issues. Our group has included a chap with one leg (who often delighted in letting new partners put an ankle lock on

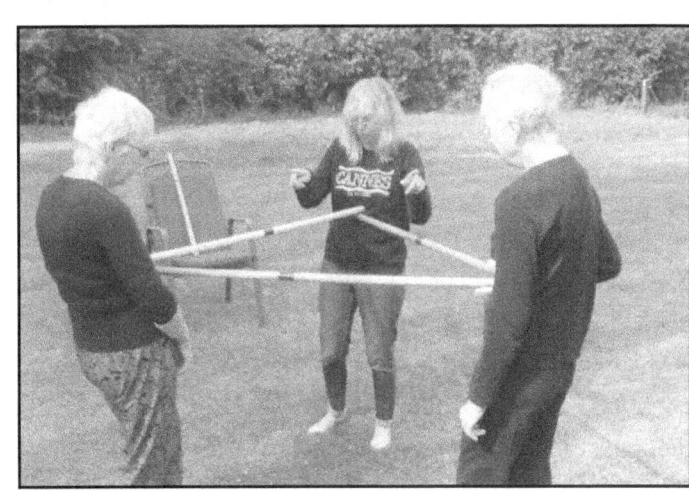

when grappling!) and a young man with autism.

It is impossible to give specific advise, but I have found the best approach is through good communication to establish both exactly what the issues are, and also what the person is seeking to get from their training. From there you can progress to adjusting the training accordingly. It may be that run an integrated class, or it may be that you run as a specific group. I do remember way back at junior school, how any disabled kids were separated out and sent to "special school." It is nice to see how these days pupils are integrated together in a much more inclusive way, and there is as much healthier approach to mental health issues too.

I recently became aware of groups such as the Adaptive Martial Arts Association who specialise in this area, so it may well be worth contacting such a group for help and advice and support.

PROFESSIONAL

On many occasions I have been invited in to teach for various organisations. I earlier mentioned teaching self defence at a local sixth form college, and have done the same for teacher groups, staff who deal with public and groups of door staff. In addition, I have taught fitness classes at various offices / workplaces and conducted specific training for close protection personnel. The point is that each case called for a specific approach to training.

In our general Systema class, we take a broad approach, covering many different aspects of training. I the teaching is more bespoke, so to speak, it needs to be focused on relevant topics. So for CP work, there will be more emphasis on awareness, communication and moving/protecting another person. Door work will cover aspects of the above, plus some control and restraint work.

In short, be sure before committing to such a class that you are a) clear about the needs of the group and, b) have the required skills to teach them. Do not feel that you have to be an expert in the particular field. For example, I don't have to be a champion race car driver to give advice on breathing in stressful conditions.

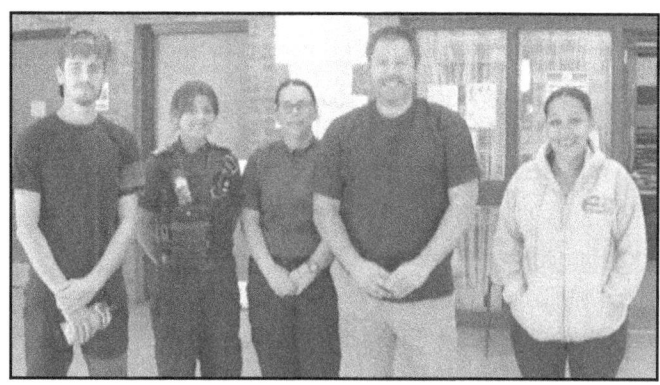

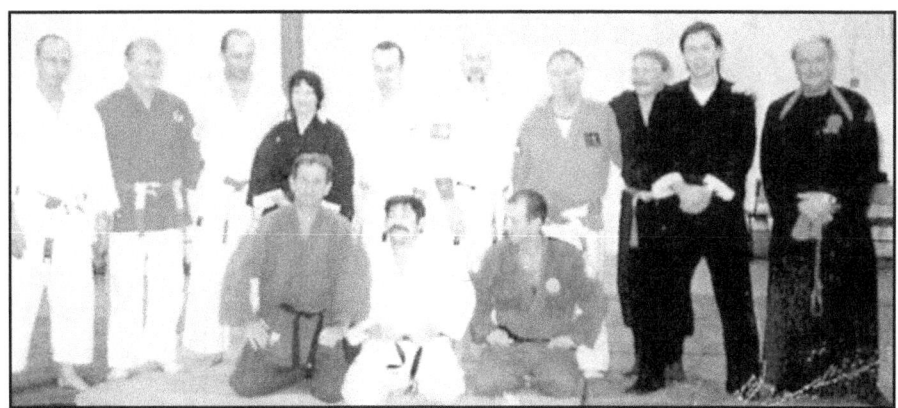

However, I won't be showing anyone how to drive!

A word when working with experts and professionals. We touched on this before but it bears repeating. I have taught many other styles of martial artists, some at high level. I've also taught experienced / special forces level military personnel. Whatever the occupation, I am careful to stay in lane and frame my work in terms of "helping you to be better at what you do," not "What I do is better than what you do."

It is always worth asking "what are you looking to get from the training." I know that this will have been discussed with the organisers, but you may not be surprised to know that the needs of management don't always coincide with the needs of staff!

Be realistic in your presentation and do not try to "impress." I ran two Knife Awareness courses for a local youth group, also with some PCSOs in attendance (volunteer police officers). When chatting with the organisers I asked why they chose me above the various other local instructors. They responded that the other instructors, on hearing that the subject was knife defence, started talking about how they would teach flashy techniques to kick the knife away, etc.

My approach was to explain how I would talk about stress management in that situation, show how knives are carried, ideas for escape and so on. In other words, the less "sexy" stuff but, by far, the most important type of work for any person faced with the potential of knife threat.

When teaching martial artists of other styles - whether they are visiting your class, or you are working at a multi-style event - you may find yourself facing different levels of "challenge." This is something I will cover in more detail later on, though I will say that if you follow the guidelines on how you present yourself, you should sidestep most issues.

CHAPTER FIVE
STRUCTURING A CLASS

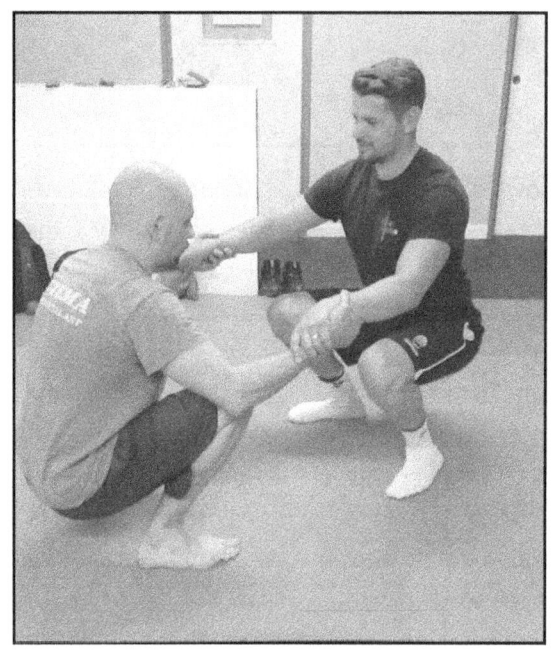

With everything in place, we can now start to look at the mechanics of teaching. If you are just starting out teaching, I suggest this procedure:

Write out a list of topics that you wish to cover in a class.
Allocate each a set amount of time according to priorities.
Allow a bit of leeway in your timings, better to have some extra time than run out halfway through a drill.

So let us say you have a regular 90 minute class, during which you wish to cover warm-up, some movement work, developing strikes, some sparring and a cool down. Your list might look like this:

Warm-up   10 minutes
Movement work – 10 minutes
Developing strikes – 20 minutes
Sparring – 30 minutes
Cool down – 10 minutes
Circle up / chat - 10 minutes

When you write the list, leave a gap between each heading. Once you have your timings, go in and fill the gaps with some specific ideas. So now we have:

Warm-up (10)
Static breathing with relax / tense
Joint rotation
Push ups, squats, leg raises, 20 of each
Movement work (10)
Dalek drill (group)
Work in pairs, evade punches (slow)
Confined area run / avoid (group)

Developing strikes (20)
Push partner with fist, placement and angle
Hitting partner
Hitting pads
Combinations / flow

Sparring (30)
Pairs sparring, varying speed
Ditto in groups of three
Ditto with whole group
Defending with strikes vs grabs
Working against boxing type attacks
Free play

Cool down (10)
Static breathing with tense / relax

There is a saying about no plan surviving contact with the enemy and the same goes for class plans! Be prepared to change or go off on a tangent if required. Students sometimes ask very good questions which might take the training of in a slightly different direction. On the other hand, you may find you need to stay on one drill for a bit longer, in order to make sure that everyone gets it.

Be wary of rushing people through drills, give them a chance for things to sink in a bit. At the same time, there is no need to drag drills out beyond a certain point. Remember, by and large we are working on student attributes rather than memorising patterns, there is little need for the endless repetition that can characterise some other martial ar styles.

Also be wary of being pushed too much off course or of pandering too much to questions that lead nowhere. Most questions should be about the specifics of the drill and most should be answerable by getting people to actually do the drill. Also be wary of "what if" questions. There is nothing wrong with these if they relate directly to the drill, but they can get quite abstract, even bizarre. My favourite, when showing work directly against the flat of a knife blade was "what if he has a light sabre?" And yes, the young lad was serious. Asking the right question is as much of a skill as being able to answer them!

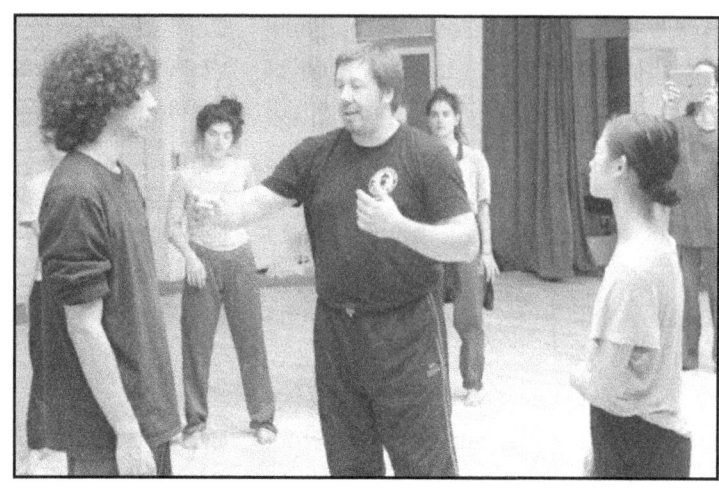

HOW MUCH SHOULD I EXPLAIN?

When people do ask questions, how should you answer them? Or, when setting up a drill or exercise, how much detail should you go into prior to starting it? Personally, I like to keep explanations brief. Outline the structure of the drill, what is required from each participant and general restrictions - speed, contact levels, etc.

You might briefly explain what the drill is for, I tend to do that as the students are actually in the drill. Time is limited, better to spend it in activity than in standing round listening. I've seen people paired with a new student start to explain the ins and outs of the drill in great detail. The poor beginner usually stands there nodding, then just as the explanation finishes, the instructor calls "switch!" so they don't get a chance to actually do the drill.

Also be wary of talking about yourself too much! I remember a workshop I went to some years back. The instructor was on his first visit to the UK and was overly keen to impress the experienced crowd with his feats of taking on biker gangs and similar tales of *derring do*. Consequently, at least half the training time was spent listening to his various exploits and "war stories." I found that it detracted from the training (which was not that great in any case) and it did nothing to boost his standing either -

in fact, he never returned to the UK despite considerable marketing (including a claim that he "taught the SAS".)

Personal experience, where relevant, is useful, of course, whether from the instructor or a student. Just be sure to keep it on point and don't use it to boost your ego. In fact, also be sure to throw in some of those times where things went wrong, they are frequently more educational!

By the way, one other interesting thing with that particular visiting instructor that I just mentioned was his use of language. He didn't just punch someone, he "f-----g punched someone." I'm far from being a prude, I swear as much as anyone. But in the setting of a group he'd never met before, with a mix of ages and types of people, it came across as crass and just part of the "I'm a real tough guy" routine. Again, this is really a social skill, or what we might call Social Systema. Read the room and pitch your tone accordingly.

That's for general classes. For workshops on specific topics, I often prepare a set of large notes or diagrams for the group to look at. These may be anatomy diagrams, a chart showing the OODA loop, scientific or bio-physical explanations and so on. In the course of the workshop I will refer to these and always make the point that further research should be conducted outside of class. We have amazing access to a world of information these days, it should be taken advantage of.

And as I mentioned, don't try and bluff it. If you don't know or aren't sure, say so – in any case you can probably get an answer off your phone in two minutes And, also as mentioned before, use the expertise of people in the group in these situations - having a Doctor or bio-mechanical engineer present can be a great help!

Another form of explanation is to use a person or people to demonstrate on. It is very important when doing this not to lose sight of the purpose of the demo. Keep it short and to the point, also, keep contact levels appropriate. I remember teaching at a multi-style workshop in Europe in the 90s. Another instructor used a young lad for his

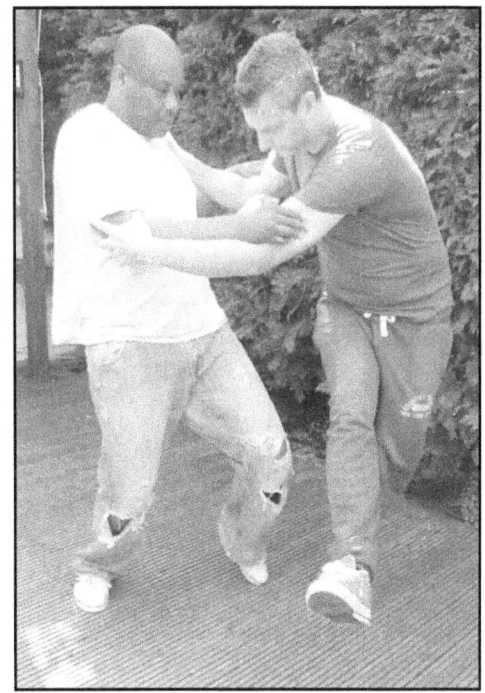

demo and absolutely flattened him on each (pre-arranged) attack. I mean really flattened him, he even kicked him square in the groin on one attack. You could hear the group groan each time and the demo seemed to go on for ever. That instructor lost a lot of respect that day and was never invited back.

It's not to say you can't hit or throw students - that is an aspect of Systema training and is something I will explain more later on - but spectators will soon pick up if you are doing so purely as an ego-boost rather than for instructional purposes.

Likewise, keep demos to an appropriate length. You should get a feel for this over time, it's a similar skill to reading a crowd for a performer. Please don't be like one guy I use to work with, whose demos went on and on, in fact people even started making a cup of tea during one - check the ego again!

In short, students should have enough prior explanation to know what is expected of them during the drill. You may or may not choose to tell them "why" before the drill, sometimes it is good to let them work it out for themselves.

The main thing is to be clear about the boundaries of the drill, then to keep an eye on things and monitor them. I will return to this subject in more detail in a later chapter.

HOW MUCH EXERCISE?

I mentioned warm ups and exercises in my example above. I have been told before "I didn't come to training to do push ups, I can do those at home!" Okay, fair enough, but.... do you,? Also what people sometimes fail to appreciate is that for us, the exercises are actually part of the "combat" training. In a way you can think of them as the Systema "kata". Push ups teach you how to punch. Squats are used when you do a take-down. Sit ups work into your ground fighting. There's a myriad other exercises and ways in which they are practically applied, let alone the actual physical / psychological benefits of doing them.

To be fair, I can understand where that guy was coming from, having been through the rather perfunctory warm ups in some

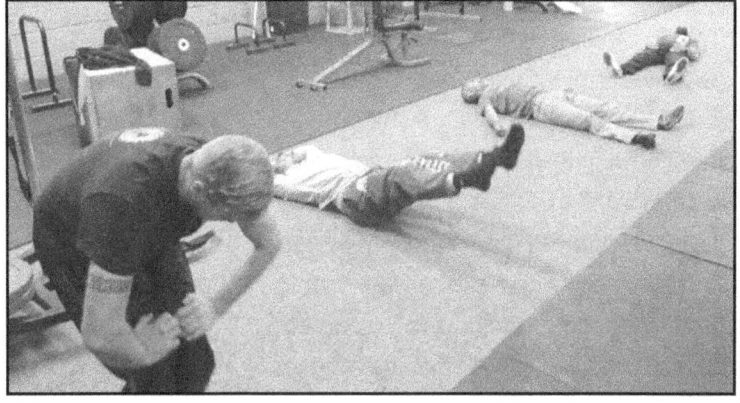

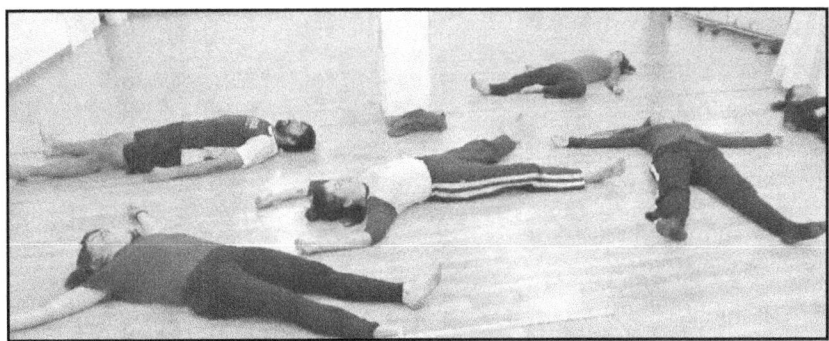

classes. At my first ever martial arts school, we went through exactly the same (not very good) exercise routine for years - in fact the class was run to exactly the same format every session. I've also attended various other sessions where the warm up is seen as a bit of a chore, something to rush through before getting on to the "good stuff." They always tended to be very similar, a bit of jumping about, some press ups and a quick stretch.

The thing is, that with the Systema approach, there is so much depth purely in the "basic" exercises, you could easily spend an hour on them (and sometimes we do.) The number of ways a simple push-up can be tweaked, practiced solo, in pairs, in fours, even, is quite remarkable. And each variation brings with it a refinement that feeds directly into our application work, whether from a structural, strength, movement, internal work, breathing or similar angle.

Having said that, with a new group, keep exercise to just what is required. We are there to teach, not entertain, but if the first class includes a 30 minute static push-up, you will have very few people coming back for Week Two! Of course, there is also a point to be made that exercises should be done outside of the class, they are a mainstay of solo training and important to overall development.

So the answer to the question is – it depends! For regular class, I like to include at least some exercise component. It prepares the body for the work and also gives you the ability to do some of the work. If you can't lift yourself up off the floor, you have little hope of surviving in grappling. Likewise, I like to tie exercise in to the practical work too, so will often show how the movement from an exercise can be directly applied against another person.

With exercise comes the question of fitness. It is always good to be fit, when not taken to some extreme or obsession. Given no health or injury issues, students should be capable of doing a reasonable amount of squats, sit-ups, push ups and of jogging around the room for ten minutes. The important thing for me - and I almost hesitate to say the phrase, so over and wrongly used has it become - is that we train *functional fitness*. Think about basic human movement. We should all be able to walk, run, crawl, climb, swim, lift things. There are seven basic movements the human body can perform and all other exercises are merely variations of these seven: Pull, Push, Squat, Lunge, Hinge, Rotation and Gait.

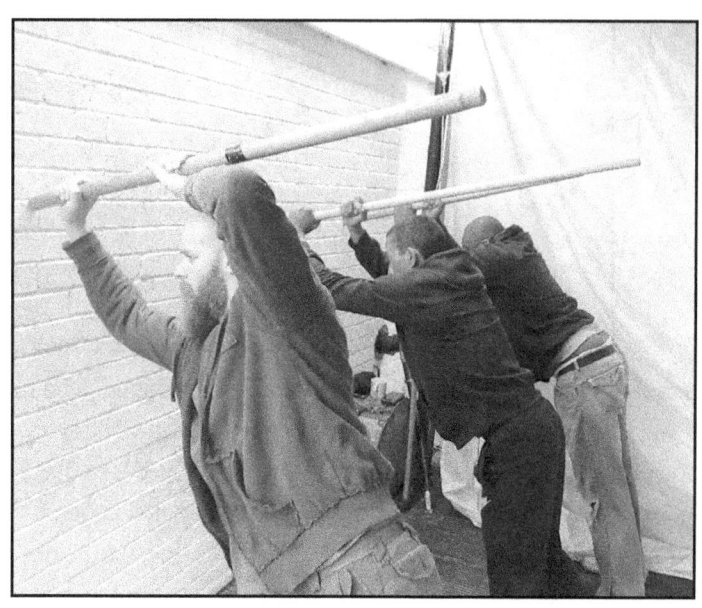

It should be easy to see how our exercises fit into one or more of these categories. Keeping an eye on function also reminds us to include a strong mobility component on our exercise.

Systema breathing adds yet another dimension to these basic human movements which, to me, takes them way beyond the "numbers" approach of a typical gym. If you explain and incorporate these concepts into the exercise /warm up phase of your class, you will find that students soon come to appreciate that phase rather than see it as a chore. I say warm-up, but another aspect of the Systema class is that you can place exercises throughout the session.

A friend of mine, when watching me teach at a workshop, said, "I noticed that you put exercises throughout the session, not just at the start, like the traditional way."

I explained the above and also how you can also use exercises to "punctuate" a class. If people need calming down, then have them do a slow push-up. If they've been doing a lot of upper body work, add in some squats. And, as mentioned, tie the exercises you've just done into the next drill sequence.

If time is short, you can also give students ideas and methods for fitness and strength training that they can go away and use. The breathing is a prime example of this. A short jog round the hall can be enough to get people into the basic square breathing method. They can then use this on longer runs in their own time.

Finally, it goes without saying that that people are in different shapes, conditions and states of injury, so any exercise must be tailored with that in mind. You may even wish to run an exercise only class - I currently run a Zoom class built purely around stick and breath-work, we have an age range of 30-75 taking part!

PACING A CLASS

The pace of your class will depend on the topics you cover and the students you have. For a new group I'd keep things moving fairly quickly, minimal explanation, with a variety of intensity. Follow a light drill with something more intense, then dial it back again, depending on how people react. Participants should leave the class feeling like they've had a work out, but also feeling energized and relaxed. It might sound contradictory, but people who have been through it will know what I mean. What I like hearing the most is when people in the circle say, "I always feel better after the class than when I came in."

Giving people just enough, physically and mentally, to challenge but not overwhelm them is a teaching skill that comes with experience. Flow state is said to be when humans are at their happiest, we will explore this idea of flow a little later.

One thing that helps with pacing is to build in a progression throughout the class based on a particular theme. Here's an example, you will see how this approach gives your class a natural structure.

Overall class theme - ground fighting.

Breathing preparation - on the floor selective tension routine, followed by static breath holds and recovery

Moving preparation - solo ground movement, starting with twisting and stretching, followed by moving with isolated body parts (eg, shoulders, legs, etc) on back, side and front.

Partner preparation - isolated movement as above, with a passive partner laying atop. Followed by movement to shift your (still passive) partner from off you.

Partner work one- A lays on floor/ B kneels next to them and must stop them getting up

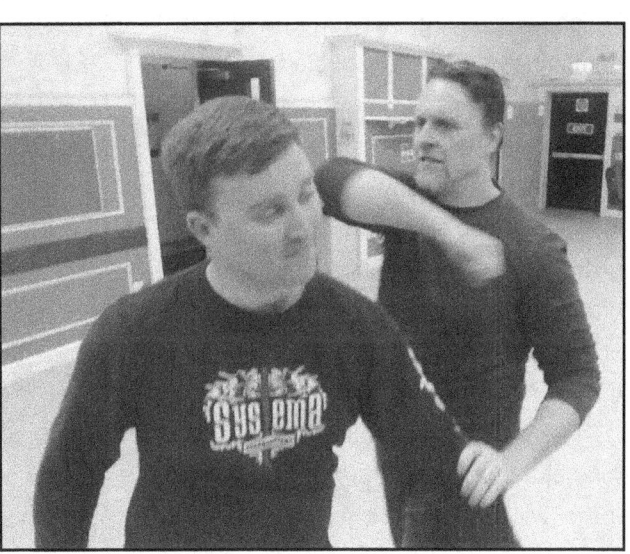

by placing hands on points of tension, breaking structure, etc. Repeat on back, sides and front.

Partner work two - take a specific technique, eg ankle lock. Show basic application followed by counters and escapes. Once they can perform the technique, partners drill apply and counter/escape.

Exercise break - press ups, sit ups, squats.

Partner work three - grab and escape drill, both on floor. Next, grab, escape and counter.

Partner work four - slow sparring, on the ground

Partner work five - pair sit back to back. On the signal they must try and subdue / submit the other, full speed. 30 seconds, then re-set. Switch partners every couple of goes.

Finish - breathing with tense and relax, stretching and twisting, circle up.

Notice how the pace of the class goes up and down. Intensity levels vary. The learning phase should be clam and quiet, giving everyone a chance to absorb and practice the information. Full speed work is preceded by slow sparring, which, in turn, is followed by a cool down.

This way, you should find the class runs at a pace suitable for all. Of course, there will be times when you wish to prolong the intensity, or even have a class that is all slow (which can be surprisingly intense in many ways.) Again, it is all down to context - who are your students, what are their training goals, what is the aim of the class., Which leads us on to our next subject.

WHAT TO TEACH?

As I have said before, Systema is great because it offers a breadth and depth of topics for learning unmatched by any other style. And, Systema is a nightmare to teach because it offers a breadth and depth of topics for learning unmatched by any other style. Where do we start?

I've already covered the different types of class you might be running, and this will largely inform your content. Seniors with a primary interest in health and movement

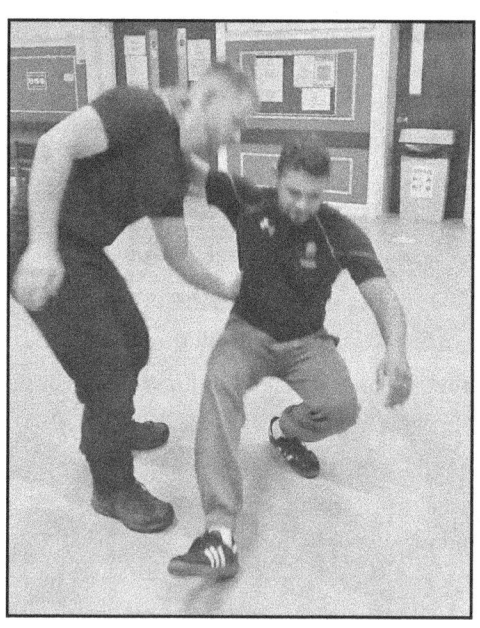

will not be so keen on working over an assault course. However, participants in a Systema camp love this type of work.

In a large part, then, it should be common sense. When you know what type of class you are offering, it's a good idea to jot down some ideas for content. This doesn't have to be a detailed syllabus, by any means. Any martial artist who has at some point set up their own school will no doubt be familiar with this.

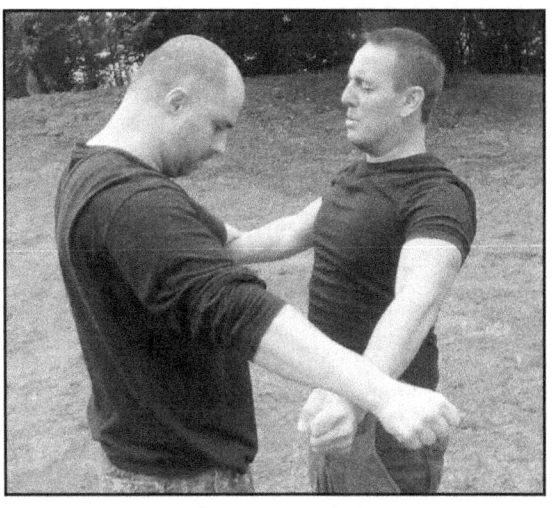

When Dave Nicholson and I set up our school CEICS (*Cutting Edge Internal Combat System*), we spent a lot of time drawing up a syllabus, adding certain topics in at certain levels, and so on. We didn't add in a grading system as such, but there was a definite progression through the levels, from basic to more advanced work.

When I got fully into Systema, that approach was largely blown out of the water! I found myself in a totally new environment where "basic" and "advanced" all trained together, where the teaching seemed curiously random, yet at the same time formed a cohesive whole. It took some time to adjust and I'm sure I made numerous mistakes on the way (and still do, learning to teach is as endless as any other type of learning.)

First, I had to decide what my teaching was *for*. To this day, it remains largely the same. The primary goal in my regular classes is to equip students with the attributes and skills necessary for "day to day" self defence.

I'll qualify that by saying that for me, self defence is a broad term that goes way beyond the confines of the average self defence class. What I tend to see in those is a total focus on the actual fight itself, that ten seconds of activity when the fists fly. To my mind, true self defence covers a much broader set of subjects. We can consider awareness, both internal and external. We can also consider after effects and consequences.

There are areas such as interpersonal skills, reading body language, knowledge of the law. Then there is the question of how we train - through constant adrenalisation which not only hampers skill development but may have negative impacts on our health? Or through a layered, cohesive approach that takes care of our bodies and minds as much as possible, while still delivering practical attributes?

I hear of so many clubs where students receive regular injuries, yet most of their training is non-contact! What sense does it make to injure yourself so much in the pursuit of protecting yourself against a probably minor incident that might never happen?

In Systema we work full contact, yet not only are injuries rare, we find that the attributes we develop map exactly and precisely onto all other activities and areas of life. This is because Systema is not a "self defence" style, it is a method of behavioural training.

This means that part of our "self defence" training incorporates massage, mobility and so on. Another primary consideration for me is that none of the training should, of itself, be harmful to the individual. Now, of course, we all get bumps and bruises from time to time. But Systema training is designed to enhance, not destroy.

My years in Taiji, for example, gave me a strong spine, but almost wrecked my knees. Even now, I cringe when I hear older martial artists say "well you just have to accept that you are going to destroy your hips doing MA." No you don't.

So, with that in place, I began thinking about all the various components that make up general self defence. Listed, they might look something like this, in no particular order.

Reasonable level of strength, mobility and fitness

Ability to deliver and defend kicks, punches, grabs and holds

Working on the ground

Working against multiples and in crowds

Working in different environments and situations

General and specific awareness

Fear and stress control

Communication skills

Working with and against day-to-day weapons.

General physical and mental health.

Opportunity to test skills.

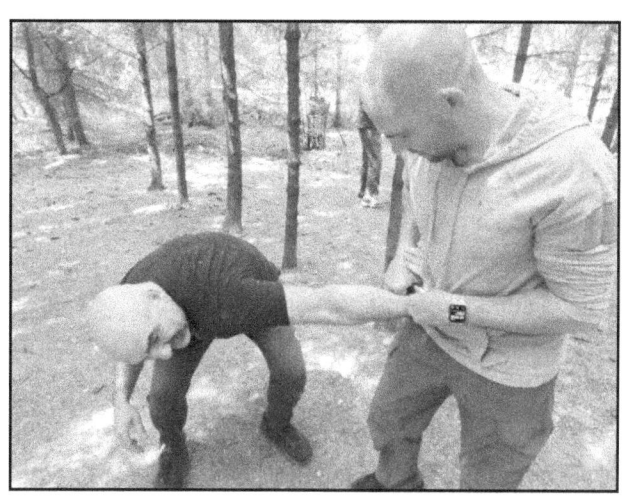

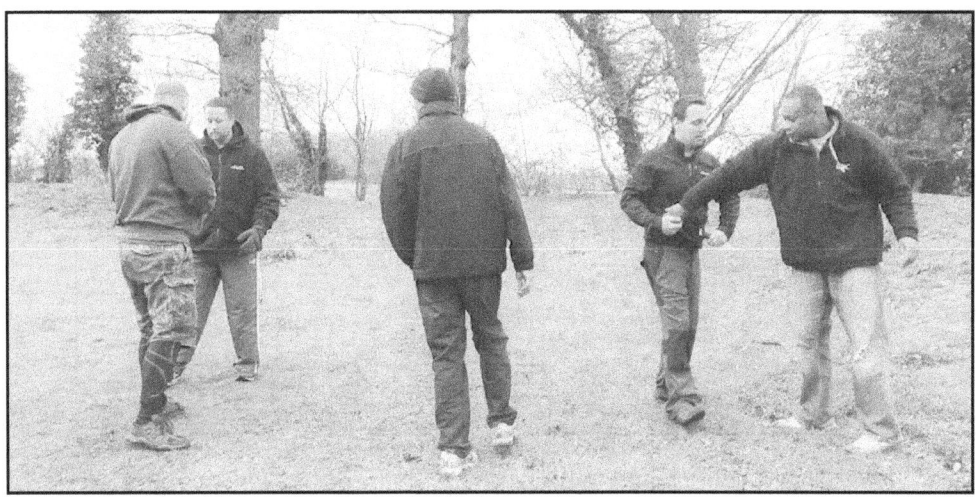

From that list it is quite easy to start mapping out a syllabus. Fear control is key, so let's start with breathing. For strength, we have all the exercises. People need to know how to manage impact, so add in falls and taking strikes. For testing skills, various types of sparring drill. And so on.

You should make it clear to prospective students what your class is for and about. Don't be tempted to mix. Having people in the "fighty" class who are interested purely in health doesn't work, in my experience. They end up sitting half the lesson out. This is not to say that you can't have elements of one in the other, but you don;t go to a French class to learn Spanish.

Above all, remember that you are in charge! I saw a post on social media recently that totally left me speechless - and that is saying something! It was by a chap in Australia who had been asked to rate Systema across various topics. When it came to realism or applicability, he gave it a low score. Why? "Because there was never any sparring in class. It was never tested."

Okay, fair enough, you might say. Here's the punchline - *that guy was the class instructor!* Dude, if you wanted to do some sparring, why not have the class, er....do some sparring?

This is another aspect of Systema - don't expect to get spoon-fed. Yes, support is always available from colleagues and the higher ups, but, surely, part of the purpose of Systema is to produce a fully functional human being. Which includes the ability to organise your class as you see fit. This issue manifested another way recently, when a new student asked if I could "write me up a training programme with all the things I need to do on it"

I said no. How it works is you come to class, I show you things, you go away and

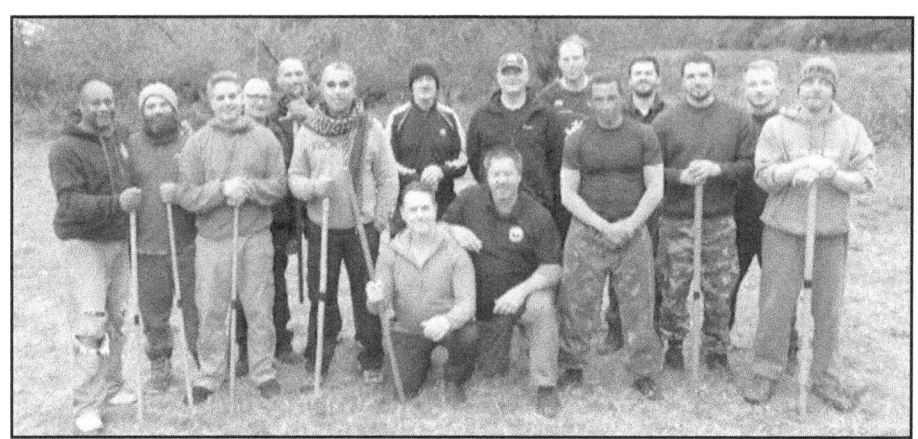

practice them. That might sound a bit harsh, but this was not a young person new to martial arts. Again, help and support is always available, but you are here to learn how to think for yourself - I hope!

How you get this across to students is up to you. I suppose I am lucky in that the vast majority of people who train with me know are either long-term regulars, who know what's what, or people with experience in the same or similar fields. They understand that this is not a gym-type situation where you tick off boxes each session.

Beginners may certainly need more of a helping hand, and this is one reason I began making DVDs and Youtube clips back in the day, to give them some form of guidance outside of class to refer to. By and large, though, you should encourage people to be self-sufficient where possible, and be direct and ready to ask for help where required.

So, back to our topic, what you teach is largely dependent on what your class is about and who it is for. Another thing to consider is that Systema is very good at teaching us the same things in several different ways. For example, given that we are breathing in every drill, then every drill is a breathing drill! This integration or holistic aspect is something that Systema excels it and is one reason we are able to all train together in the same class. Consider the simple push-up as an example. Here, we have five people all doing push-ups. Ah, right, all doing the same thing, you might think. But look closer.

Andy is blasting through the push-ups, inhale down, exhale up, working hard and fast.

Tracy is concentrating on her form, keeping the back perfectly level as she raises and lowers. The breathing is helping her with this.

John is working to minimise tension

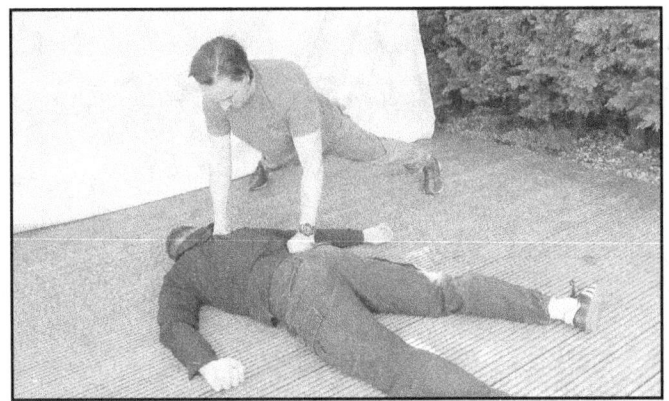

throughout the body. Just a little in the fists, he is trying to see if he is relaxed enough to rotate his shoulders as he goes up and down.

Aisha is in the flow, keeping the breathing smooth, in total co-ordination with the movement

Ben is struggling, his fists hurt on the floor, his breath is sporadic, he can barely do five push ups.

Same exercise, five people, five different experiences. Now apply that across the whole spectrum of Systema training and you can being to see how this integration of people and practice works.

What this means for the Instructor, is that you can often drop in a sneaky breathing drill disguised as, say, work with the focus pads. Halfway through, have everyone take an in breath and hold. Not only are the students now getting the biomechanics of the strikes working, they are also learning to deal with discomfort and stress, and also how to recover while on the move.

But what if you find yourself short of idea? Maybe you have a few favourite drills, but want to add in some variations. Training with main teachers where you can is an obvious source of fresh ideas, but also consider how fortunate we are nowadays with the overwhelming amount of information we have at our fingertips.

When I first started martial arts training there were literally two books in the local library (one on Karate, one on Judo) and maybe one or two magazines, that you could often only get in martial art shops.

So these days, you should never be short of ideas for a class. A quick browse of "Systema" on Youtube will give you plenty, and don't be afraid to "borrow" from other styles, either, or even other activities. I picked up some great reaction drills from a tennis channel, for example. You might even throw it open to the class. Ask people what they want to do, and see what ideas they come up with - they might surprise you!

CHAPTER SIX
MANAGING A CLASS

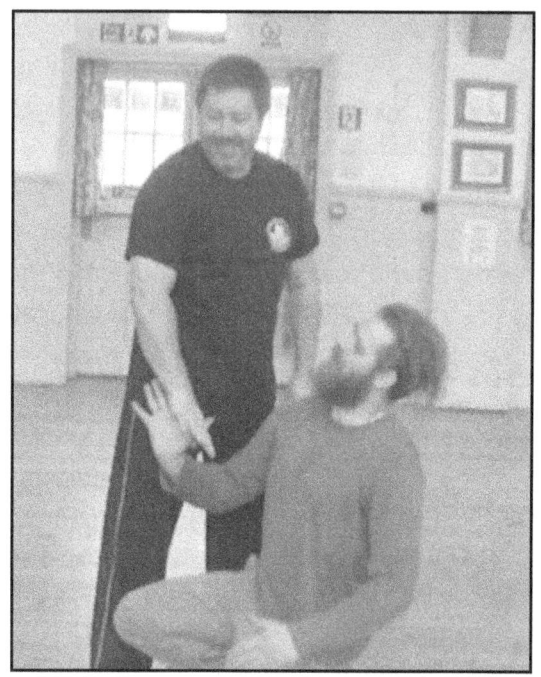

Setting up and running drills is only one aspect of teaching. As an instructor you needs to be constantly aware of what is going on in class and how to deal with any issues that arise. As with most teaching, we need to go beyond the core skills of our particular subject and into the realms of communication, people management, even counselling at times. So let us look at some of the issues you may encounter while teaching and suggest some ways to pre-empt or manage them.

There are two things to do before training starts. You should make it clear that participation in any drill is optional. Everyone has the right to sit out something they feel is not for them, without any judgement from the group. You should also ask if people have any particular injury or condition that needs to be taken into account. If it is a new group I will also spend a few minutes discussing what we are going to do and emphasising that people should always train safely.

LEARNING STYLES

When outlining drills and exercises be as clear, precise and concise as possible. As an aid to this, you might like to consider the theory of Learning Styles. This became popular in the 1970s, to the point of eventually spawning somewhere around 71 different models!

To a large extent, the theory has more recently fallen out of favour. In fact, since 2012, learning styles have often been referred to as a "neuromyth" in education. However, there are some aspects of Learning Styles that you might find useful as a starting point, without having to get too wrapped up in the theory. If nothing else, they may give you some thoughts on how you present your material.

We will look at two theories. The first is Neil Fleming's VARK model, which expanded upon earlier notions of sensory modalities. The four sensory modalities in Fleming's model are:

Visual learning
Aural learning
Reading/writing learning
Kinesthetic learning
Multimodality (MM)

While the fifth modality isn't considered one of the four learning styles, it covers those who fit equally among two or more areas.

Fleming claimed that visual learners have a preference for seeing. They respond well to visual aids such as graphs, charts, diagrams, etc. In Systema terms, this person benefits more from watching a drill or movement being demonstrated.

Auditory learners prefer to learn through listening. So they respond best to verbal explanations and detailed instruction.

Reading/writing is quite self explanatory, though less applicable to the average Systema class.

Finally, kinesthetic learners prefer to learn via experience - moving, touching, and doing, what we might call active exploration. Fleming's model also posits multi-modality. This means that not everyone has one defined preferred modality of learning; some people may have a mixture that makes up their preferred learning style.

You might like to consider your own experience, and speak to your students about this to see if any of them express a preference. Sometimes it can be quite apparent. I sometimes find, when demonstrating a drill, that some people pay rapt attention to what I am doing, while others are glancing round the room, seemingly paying little attention. It is not unusual for the latter to then ask, as we go into the drill, "what are we doing?" It is as though they need the exercise fully explained to them verbally.

Personally, I've always found that I can pick things up quite well visually. I see a movement and have a good go at replicating it. Years back, I trained some classical Ju Jitsu, where the instruction was very verbal. "Place your left foot here, your right hand goes there." I always found it a struggle to retain that information. So while the theory has fallen out of flavour, there may be something to be said for it, at least as a general framework for starting out.

Be sensitive as to how people are reacting to the information you're giving out. We've already spoken about keeping explanations and demos to an appropriate length. You might also experiment with presenting the same drill in three different ways. First, talk and explain. Then demo with a partner. Finally, guide students through it tactiley, actually move them into position.

Now, onto our second Learning Styles theory, which takes a more cognitive approach. In 1974 Anthony Grasha and Sheryl Riechmann, formulated the Grasha-Reichmann Learning Style Scale. This was developed to analyse the attitudes of students and how they approach learning, in order to provide teachers with insight on formulating instructional plans for college students. The names of Grasha and Riechmann's learning styles are:

Avoidant - tend to perform poorly, are unenthusiastic about learning, do not engage with other students or teachers Absenteeism is often a problem with avoidant learners. Exams and tests do not suit avoidant learners, they prefer a more relaxed teaching style

Participative - engage with their teachers and relate well to peers. They are good at

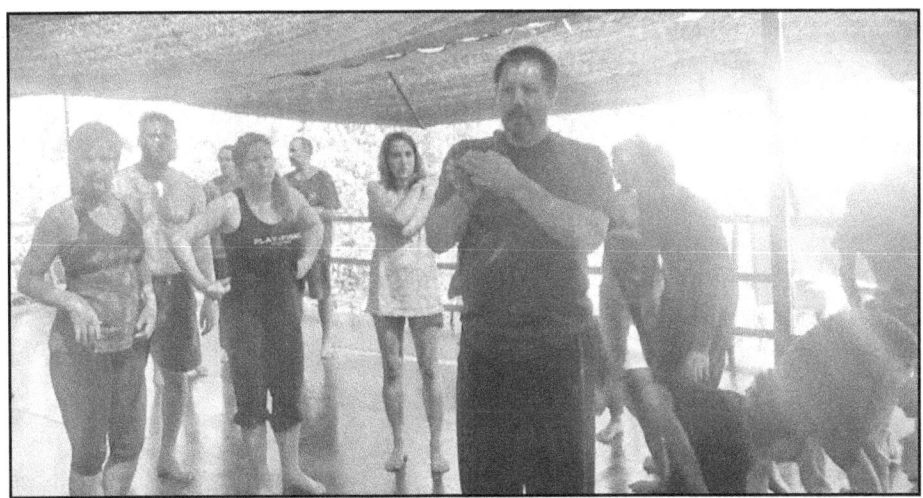

accepting responsibility for their own work and like to make the most of all learning situations. Participative learners enjoy getting involved, preferring to be directly involved in the class rather than being asked to listen to a lecture in silence.

Competitive - prioritise learning as a way to outperform other students in their class. They feel their only reward is to outstrip the competition.

Collaborative - work best in harmony with their peers and blossom as part of a team. Respond well to team projects.

Dependent - dislike change, tend to learn only what is required to get by, and become frustrated if they are asked to explore ideas that are not fully explained. Prefer clear outlines, notes and instructions, following the teacher, and avoiding ambiguity.

Independent - relish the opportunity to think for themselves. Will often work outside of the curriculum if they feel a topic deserves further exploration. Whilst they prefer to work alone, they are also good as part of a team, and will listen to the ideas of their peers.

Bear in mind that these categorisations were formulated specifically for college students, but I think there is some application here for Systema classes too. We might see "avoidant" students as those who attend class infrequently, even though they may have paid for it. It might be akin to the "New Year gym membership" syndrome where people, with the best intentions, pay an annual gym fee, yet only attend a few sessions. Some studies put this figure as high as 67%! It is why gyms adopt the annual fee model, without those people they would go bust!

It is less common to find annual charges in

martial art classes (though not totally unknown.) However, even on the standing order model, you will find people who pay per month yet very rarely turn up. In fact, I had one person who carried on paying for two years without attending!

There may be reasons for this. Circumstances may change and people forget to cancel the SO. People want to continue supporting the group even if they can't attend. People get out of the habit of coming to class but feel that by still paying, they continue to be involved in the club.

As an instructor, you have to recognise that you are in a minority. Very few people, especially now, commit to even a weekly class with diligence and enthusiasm. This doesn't just apply to martial arts. I was surprised some years back when, on taking an evening class, how many people paid for the course yet only attended only one or two sessions. In fact, barely a quarter of people actually got through the whole course which was only six weeks in any case!

Can we take steps to address this issue? One way is to keep in regular touch with students. This can be done via social media (I find WhatsApp works well) and/or a regular newsletter - you can run these free through Mailchimp or similar. Every ten days or so I put out an e-mail with a video clip, details of classes, workshops, discount codes for downloads, etc. This, hopefully, acts as a reminder that classes are on-going!

You might run social events for students. These could be as simple as a post-class drink, or Christmas meals, outings, etc.

Some martial art clubs will send out birthday greetings to students, or have a "Student of the Month" scheme going. Personally, I find these better suited to children's classes, but they may be something to consider.

If you haven't seen a regular student for a while, you might drop them a line, just to ask if everything is okay. People don't always want to bring their problems to class, be they bereavement, injury, illness, change in circumstances, etc. Be aware that there is a fine line between checking up on people

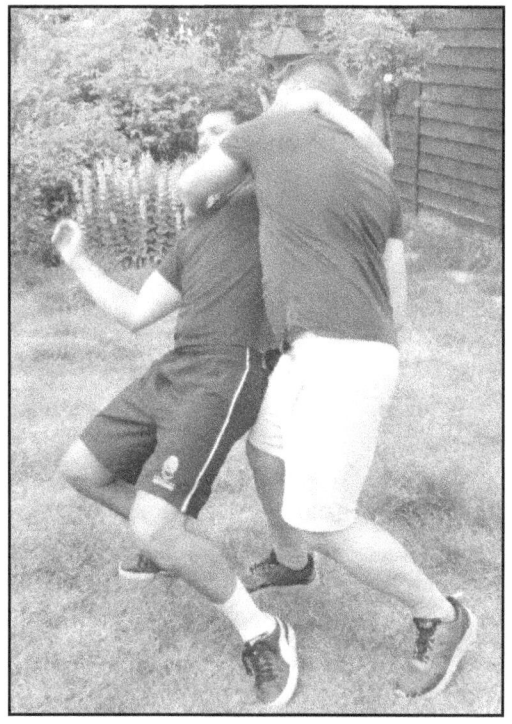

and chasing them - you don't want to sound desperate!

Every now and then I bump into a student I haven't seen for a while when out and about. Without doubt, they always say "oh the classes are great, I really miss them! I'll be back soon!" And, almost always without doubt, they never return. I usually smile and nod, it's up to the individual what they do.

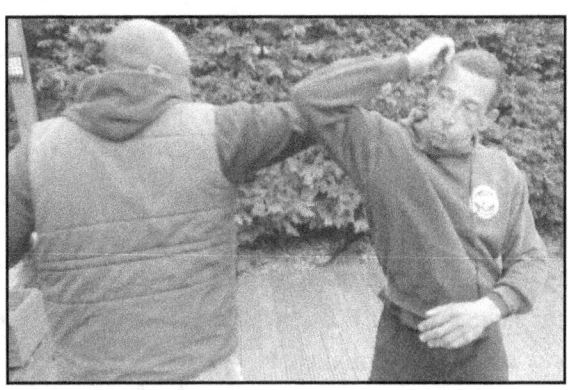

If you do bump into a person that has left, it might be useful to ask them why. I find in general that, in the UK at least, people are rarely forthcoming with complaints. However it can be a good thing to know. In one case, I found that a person had felt intimidated by another student for example, something I was not aware of at the time. There may be other issues which can only be addressed if you know about them.

None of us is above constructive criticism, though it's not something you often see in the martial arts. I feel this is largely a cultural issue. I mentioned how in certain traditions, to question the Master's authority is seen as poor form. That was certainly the environment I came up in, even once being told that "Sifu is more important than your own father!" Personally, I find this approach unhealthy and an anathema to personal development, but each to their own.

On the one hand, an instructor needs to be approachable and open to question, on the other hand, you are in charge and people are coming to you to learn. I find if you teach Systema well, everything will balance itself out in that respect. Again, it largely depends on what sort of class you are running and peoples' reasons for attending. And sometimes, at the end of the day, we have to accept that this is just the way things are.

MUTUAL BENEFIT

The "competitive" student can be an issue in class. A certain amount of "drive" is required in any martial arts training, but Systema is not really an art designed for "winning" or dominating others to fuel our ego. In fact, Systema is, as my colleague Ed Phillips often likes to say, an art where "the cheap shot" is easily applied.

An instructor must be very firm in explaining that for regular class drills, the aim of the drill is not to defeat the aim of the drill! A simple example would be a groundwork drill, where one partner says "yeah but you have to get me on the ground first!" So now it is not a groundwork drill, it is a takedown drill.

I had one student who was extremely strong, a big, powerful guy. In one to one drills, especially grappling, he could dominate almost everyone in the group. However, he often achieved this by ignoring anything that didn't hurt or injure him. In other words, fingers touching his eyes, a little tap to the groin, even, during one session, being stabbed repeatedly with a training knife.

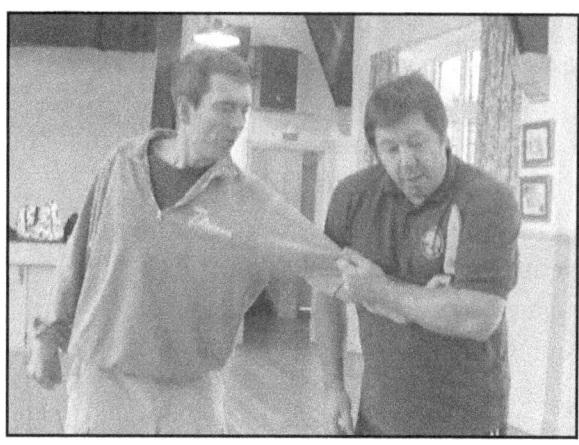

I found one way to get round this was to run multiples drills, to take that one-on-one duelling mentality away. He also became a good person to use for team work - in other words, a pair or group of three trying to restrain him. It was a shame, in a way, I could see he was learning little himself, but became used more and more as a kind of test for others - even just a simple grab and escape drill could turn into an exercise in survival. Despite repeated explanations he just couldn't let go of this idea that every drill was about totally dominating the other person, regardless of what was happening.

It was also interesting to note that he hated taking strikes - in fact he was less good at that than most of the other people. It was almost as though there was a fear of being seen as vulnerable, perhaps hence the aggression.

He eventually left the group, it was all very amicable, he told me I was "not teaching enough technique," which is fair enough. The class was not what he wanted, though perhaps it was something he needed.

So one way to deal with the overly competitive is to strictly enforce the limits of the drill. Fully explain the purpose, ie to train a particular attribute, to try out a certain principle and so on.

Another is to work less in pairs and more in threes or a group. In a free for all whole group melee, there is little scope for being competitive. Everyone gets hit.

You might also consider running some team drills, where people have to co-operate to problem solve, too. Running these at the start of the class can develop a calmer atmosphere for the rest of the session.

There is also the option of taking the wind out of a person's sails. Vladimir and Mikhail are masters at this. They both are able to easily control a person and subdue them without danger to themselves or the other person. This also relates to the subject of the "challenger" in class and I will go into more detail on this later in the chapter.

Something else to stress, unique to Systema in my experience, is the concept that both partners get something out of a drill. This is an idea totally inbuilt into Systema that stands in stark contrast to the more usual "attacker/defender" role.

In much of my early pre-Systema training, my role as "attacker", whether it be to the Sifu or a fellow student, was to feed in the required attack to the required target. It was then usually the done thing to freeze in place while the "defender" carried out his techniques.

Now, there can be a place for this, but it is not really how Systema works. First of all, we have to look at the purpose of the drill. Let's take this as an example: *A is to approach B and grab them. B allows the grab to come on almost fully, before responding with a takedown, into a control position.*

So you will note the first difference is there is no set attack other than "to grab." It might be a headlock, a bear hug, a double leg takedown. Likewise, the instruction to the other partner is "takedown and control", no specific technique is mentioned.

Here's the next thing, who is the attacker and who is the defender? There is an in-built assumption in most martial arts of good guy/bad guy. I'm initiating the attack, so I'm the villain. There are many other inherent assumptions in that, mostly based around the notion that the hero will always "win" because that's what happens in the movies, right?

But consider this situation - you are security staff or similar and there is a punter that needs restraining. You move him to grab him and he takes you to the floor. *What! This has never happened before, I'm the good guy!"*

Taking that aspect out of the Systema drill gives both participants the opportunity to experience and learn from a particular situation. Why? Because this is real life, Systema is rooted in professional work, often under the most trying of circumstances. It goes way beyond basic "attack and defend" routines into behavioural levels, where roles may not be so clearly defined as the conventional martial art setting.

Instead, then, of framing the drills as "you attack him with a grab, you respond with a take-down, " try this/

"Here's the drill. B is going to let A apply a grab. Imagine you;ve been caught by surprise, you don't see the grab coming or have time to avoid it. Before the grab fully tightens, I want you to *respond* by shifting your body structure and taking B down to the floor. B, if you feel the takedown working, then look at how you can best manage your fall to not only minimise impact, but get the best position you can on the ground.

A, when you drop the person, see if you can do it in such a way that you can control them with your knees, locking there arm, etc.

I want you to work steady, especially if you haven't done much falling before. For those who can fall well, you can begin to pick up speed once you are into the drill. No strikes at all, we're just working structure and position to help you understand how to smoothly get a person down, and also how to manage that fall. Okay, in pairs, let's go."

You can back up this explanation with a short physical demo, for the benefit of your "visual" learners. Choose one of the "kinetic" learners as your partner.

Each partner now has a clearly defined goal and framework. Of course, there are many variables to add in, which we will talk about later on. But overall, hopefully this removes us beyond the, "you grab his wrist, you apply a reverse wrist lock" approach. We are already building an element of aliveness and unpredictability into the work.

Naturally, as an instructor you are observing everything that is going on in the class all the time! Be aware if a person is becoming overly dominant with their partner. Now, as we all train in together, you might have a significant mis-match of skill levels in a pair. There are two ways to work around this.

The first is that the more experienced partner works gently and carefully, encouraging their partner as they go. The second is to give the more experienced person some kind of restriction. For example, they may only use one arm, or have eyes closed. This will do something to redress the balance and also keep things fresh and challenging for the experience student.

I do believe that this dualistic view of training has been responsible for much of the negativity directed towards Systema on social media. The prime example is seeing the teacher hit or throw the apparently totally passive student and assume that the teacher is showing off. "Won't work in real life," is the usual comment. But this is real life. They are real hits and real throws. The reason the student is passive is because the focus of the exercise is not the teacher, but the student.

We hit people to teach them how to deal with hits. We throw them to teach them how to deal with throws. The impact, the mechanics, the fear. The better at each, the more live our training can become. In other words, this is training attributes, it is not a little recreation of a fight. Again, it's training, not a movie scene for entertainment.

No-one tells a boxer that running a

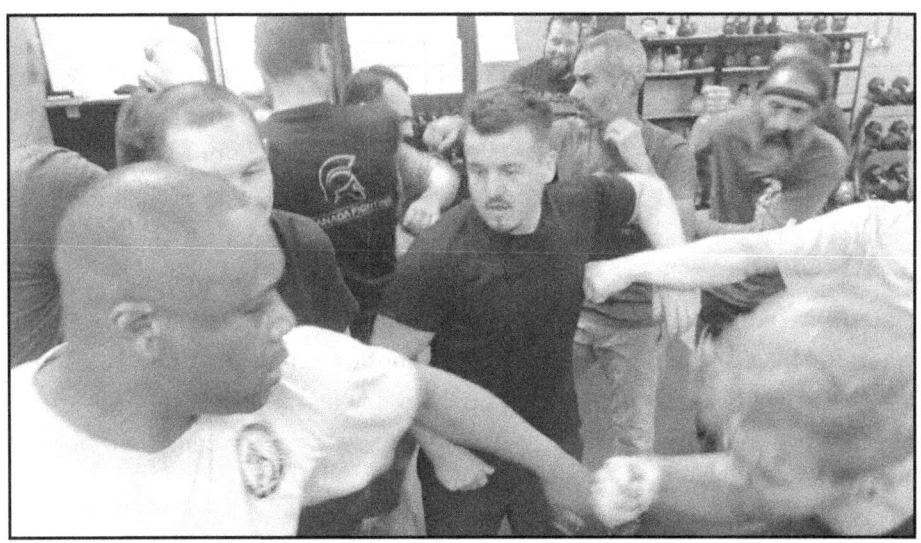

couple of miles won't work in the ring. People understand the purpose. When it comes to martial arts it seems many have been conditioned into seeing everything a a fight simulation and respond accordingly. Sometimes I am sure the poster understands this and is just dog-whistling to the crowd for Youtube hits - but that's another issue!

Is there any place for competition in Systema training? Yes, but at appropriate times and in appropriate ways. Let's look at a goal based sparring drill as an example. A has one minute to get B out of the room through a doorway. In other words, the type of situation you might find yourself in if you are door staff and have to eject an unruly customer.

In this case, B is entirely within their rights to resists all attempts by A to move them! We can still attach parameters of course - perhaps no striking or biting. But in one sense this is now a competition between A and B to each perform a specific task. The important thing is, again, how you frame it. I like to present it this way - each person is providing the other with the right conditions to test an aspect of their skill set. It is not a total simulation, as in an actual event there will be many other factors at play. However, it does help test some of the skills required to either move someone who needs moving, or resist a person who is trying to move you somewhere against your will.

The time limit is also important. It ensures that people get involved in the drill rather than bounce around each other for three minutes with barely a punch, something I see in a lot of "sparring" clips online. In order to test skills, we need people to actually engage.

So, we shift the competition away a little from "can I beat the other person?" to "can I rise to the challenge and successfully complete the task?"

The issue here is partly ego, though none of us can function without an ego. It is more a question of how we contain the ego and control it rather than have it control us. This is a very, very important lesson. I recently saw CCTV footage of a young man stabbed and killed because he chased a man with a knife who was backing away, purely out of ego. His pride resulted in his death.

Good Systema training should do much to overcome this trait, especially with it's emphasis on enduring rather than "winning." I've also found that ego-based competitiveness is an insurmountable barrier to learning anything beyond the most basic aspects of training. You simply can't get into the deeper levels without learning to "let go" at some point

There is another element of the "competitive" student and that is where the student competes with the instructor. Not on direct challenge level but in terms of "improving" the drill.

I've had it happen where the drill is set up, away we go, then a person might say to their partner, "this isn't realistic enough, let's add in this or that." When I hear this (and I hear everything in class!) I normally stop and make two points.

First, how real do you want it? Think about that for a moment. Seriously.

Second, I'll explain again the function of the drill, adding that, yes, we can add in this and that, but this is our start point. Was your first driving lesson on a motorway at rush hour? No. My first was in quiet back street, a stationary car, turning a cardboard steering wheel!

You might find that some people think they are "tougher" than the drill, it is beneath them. That may be a good time to switch into an exercise break. Thirty count press-ups, squats, sit ups, followed by a run round the hall, going to ground when I clap. That usually calms people down a bit.

It might also be that the person thinks they are helping out by tweaking the drill, along the lines of the "over-explainer" we mentioned earlier. I once saw Vladimir in this situation. He stopped the class and said to

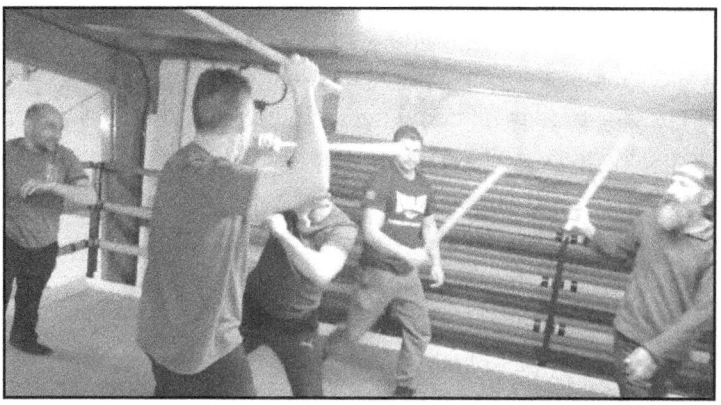

the person, "who is the instructor here, me or you?" Point made and the session continued. So treat any case of this as it needs to be treated. A gentle word, a switch in drills, putting the person in their place and so on.

That leaves the remainder of our learning types. I guess that "participative" etc students are our ideal. Keen, perceptive, willing to get involved and committed to learning. These will form the core of your regular training group and should be nurtured. These are likely the instructors of tomorrow.

RELAX!

Let's go back to the topic of how much to explain but also look at *how* we explain it. The single most common word you will hear in Systema classes is *relax*. But what does it mean? How do we achieve it? Why do we want to?

Let's begin with how we explain it. If there is one thing I can guarantee, it is that commanding people to RELAX! RELAX! Will only tense them up. The first thing, then, is to look at how we get relaxation across. Just saying "relax" on its own will not cut it, at least not with new students. Picture it - here I am in the deadly martial arts class and this person is telling me to relax. *What, like sitting by the pool with a drink and a book? By having a snooze?*

On the other hand, some people get quite indignant when you tell them to relax, they often snap back, "I am relaxed!"

Think back to our first set of Learning Styles. Regardless of the science behind them, let's use them as a framework to hang our "relaxation" on. First off, I will explain that Systema works through relaxation. That means not being completely noodle-like, but getting rid of any excess tension in the body.

Visually, I am presenting myself in a relaxed way. This is important. I have seen instructors become very "breathy" and obviously nervous in some situations. This is not likely to instil relaxation in students. We all feel nervous at times, that's fine. However, as an instructor you should be able at least to prevent that becoming outwardly obvious. If not, it is an area you need to work on. So present yourself in a calm, relaxed way and you are already setting a good visual example for your class to follow.

Onto the most important area, the kinetic or feeling. Relaxation is a state of feeling, we can't understand it only through words, we need to experience it. This is one reason that at the start of almost every session, I run through the breathing with selective tension drill. In case you don't know it, I will detail it quickly here.

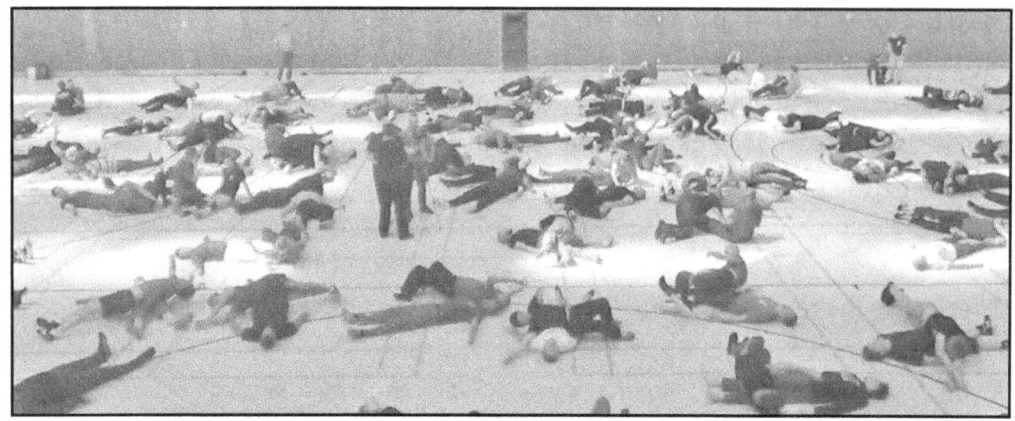

Students sit or lay down (the latter is better but not everyone wants to get on the floor straight away.) You quietly instruct them as follows:

Inhale nose, exhale mouth. Settle into your breathing, it doesn't have to be too deep. Just feel the air coming in and out of the body.

Let them settle in for a minute or two, then: On your next inhale, tense both legs fully. Just the legs, the rest of the body stays relaxed. So, long breath iiiiiiiinnn. Now, equal breath and relax, ooooout.
Repeat three times for the legs, then work abdomen, back, chest, arms, head. Then to finish:
Slow inhale again, this time tense the whole body..... And hold.   Slow exhale and hold.
Repeat three times, then have them breathe normally without tension . From there you can work into some stretching / ground movement type work.

This drill has two effects. One, it calms everyone down in readiness for the class. They may have had a hectic day and rushed in, this literally gives them a breathing space.

Two, it directly gives the person the experience of accumulating and releasing the tension. Hopefully, as that full tension is released, it takes and residual tension away with it.

This state can then be referenced later on, during a drill, for example. "Remember how you released that tension at the start? Do the same here. Exhale as you move, letting the tension go to free up the body."

Now the student has a concrete grasp of what "relax" means. Once that is established, we can work into deeper levels.

If people are still struggling, or to reinforce the concept, you can try this. At one gym we used, the walls were lined with punch bags. I told the class to "fire yourselves up, get tense and aggressive and hit the bags as hard and fast as you can. Go!"

I timed it. The longest one lasted about a minute, and there were some fit people in the class. Next I told them "now relax, use your figure eight or wave moment, hit with power, fast as you can."

This time I called a halt at three minutes, there were still people punching. It makes it quiet clear, again in a very tangible way, that excess tension hinders our movement and reduces our endurance. This is common knowledge, right? Everyone knows this - no-one expects an expert in anything to be other than relaxed. Swimmers, runners, artists, after dinner speakers, any field you can think of. Yet when it comes to martial arts, because of the perceived "toughness" or perhaps because of fear, we encounter so much tension in people.

Other ways to do it might be to ask people to perform simple tasks - even walking - while remaining fully tense. Anything that gives that experience of tension release equals freedom to move. Once that internal feedback state is established, we can move onto areas such as mindset and flow.

In short, where possible, when describing anything that involves a level of internal communication or awareness, present the information verbally, visually and, most importantly, via direct experience. Stress how much of Systema is based on feel and intuition and how that once we have established a particular internal state, we are able to drop into it much easier in the future. If you have never eaten apple pie, you cannot describe what it tastes like!

INTENSITY

Once training is underway you need to watch out for several things and will soon develop eyes in the back of your head! You need to be aware of how people are responding to the work particularly to the intensity of the drill. It may be that they are becoming a little excited and going over the required level, or it may be they are too uncomfortable with the intensity.

In the first case, we've already covered some ideas. In the second, there are times when people need to be pushed beyond their comfort limits, but this should be done in a way that is constructive and not counter-productive. This is something you will develop with experience, but as a

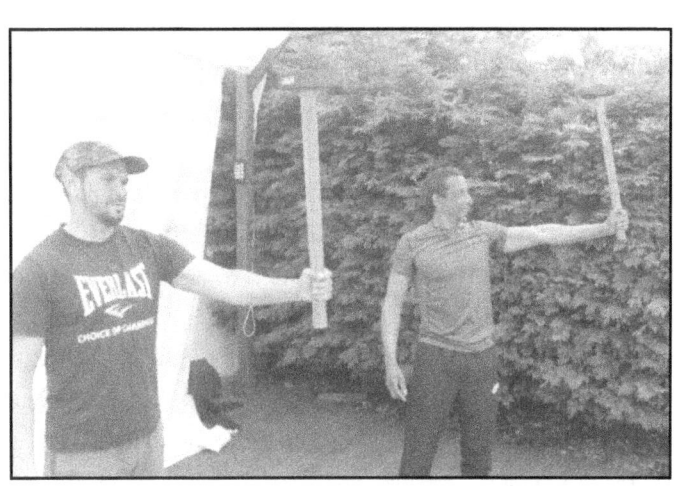

general guide if people seem very nervous then they should be led gradually into intense work. The vital thing is that you give the student a good coping mechanism in order to deal with the stress they will encounter. Too often I see people in some training methodologies being "adrenalised" but being giving no guidance as to how to deal with it other than "put your head down and fight". This means that the stress remains within the person after training and can have an increasingly negative effect over time.

Most of the time you will be monitoring that people remain within the boundaries of the drill, as well as giving any necessary guidance. Sometimes I will stop a drill to pick up on a particular mistake or point for the whole group. Also, if a pair is showing some very good work, we may stop and let the whole group watch them for a while – it is good to give positive reinforcement.

Where work is particularly intense, be sure to give clear instructions, as mentioned and, in the case of testing and scenario work, put in a time limit. Where the work is intense exercise, bear in mind that endurance levels, both physical and mental, will vary across the group. We often have to strike a balance across the group as a whole, though be careful not to pander too much to the lowest common denominator. It is interesting to see the little tricks and tactics people use to excuse themselves from intense work. I've used a few myself so now how to spot most of them. Here's a few examples:

Injury

The person steps out, often with a little grimace, always making a noise and clutching some part of their body. "Oh, it's my old elbow injury," they might say, even if we are doing duck walks. Of course, there are people with genuine injuries, but this is something that should be covered already, at the start of the class. If someone has bad knees, I'm not going to make them duck walk for ten minutes. So it may be that while the rest of the class do that, I'll get them to do some slow, assisted squats off to the side.

Likewise, it is good to encourage people to work around injuries, where possible. Following a punch gone wrong, I've had my hand taped up for a few weeks. That means no push-ups on the knuckles, so I've gone back to the flat palm in class. Not so good, but at least I'm getting some push-ups in.

Need a drink

We all know the importance of hydration but, medical issues aside, you can do without a glug of water for ten minutes. It's easy enough to work water breaks into a session, if required. I rarely do, students take a quick sip as and when they need it. I find I rarely do, besides, sometimes it's good to train when thirsty, or hungry or tired. Plus you can find that a quick ten second water break

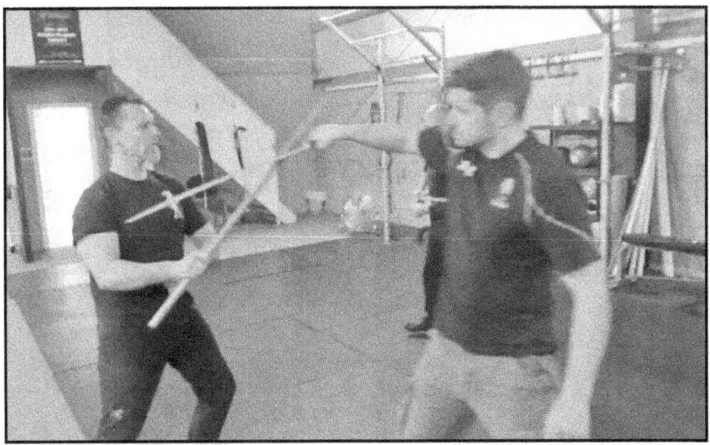

gradually morphs into a five minute break with a chat. Keep an eye on that. Speaking of which…

Need a chat
The person initiates a conversation, maybe about the exercise, more often some reminiscence of they time they, etc, etc. If you can move and talk at the same time, fine. If not, unless there is an urgent need, stop talking and get on with it. The same applies for between exercises, watch out for the "between drill chatterbox" who can slow the pace of the whole sessions.

I'm a bit tired
Yes, I know. That's why you need to do the exercises, in order to be not so tired in the future.

Where possible, I like to do the exercises alongside students. At the very least, I won't put people through something I haven't at least tried myself. There are some exercises I'm terrible at - pull ups, for example. However, it's good to lead by example where you can. I remember being told by a prominent UK martial artist that a particular exercise is "impossible to do." It's where one person stands upon another's feet as they lay on the floor. That person then stands up, I can't remember the proper name for it. So we always take delight in doing that one, I always see that sort of comment as a challenge. Like I said, we all need a bit of ego!

In short then, constantly monitor how people are coping, don't be afraid to increase or drop intensity as required and don't feel that you have to constantly go full blast every session. The ability to change gear goes down as well as up. For more personally intense work, we put a safe word in place. This is where we are working more situational rather than a straight drill or exercise. That may be in a scenario or it may be in various types of testing. In those cases, as soon as a student says the safe word, they are out of the drill - no judgement, no delay.

Of course, afterwards you can discuss this with them to find out why they stopped.

It may be that the drill triggered the memory of a particular event, it may be that the fear overwhelmed them, and so on. In no case should you force people just to "tough it out," at least in regular training beyond, their perceived limit. Military training is not always applicable to civilian life, though options are there for those who wish to push beyond the usual levels.

MINDSET

What is happening inside the brain is just as important, maybe even more so, than our physical movements. People in martial arts have varying views of what is a good mindset.

The more combative groups tend to (though not always) work from a mindset of pure aggression. I've seen some call this "feral mind, " the imagery used is often of a ferocious predator, the guard dog as opposed to the "sheep" around them.

This is a mindset that plays well to the general public and looks good in video clips and demos. Unfortunately, it's use in real life is somewhat limited - usually because it is accompanied by a lot of physical tension which, as we said before, actually hinders our movement. Furthermore, continued exposure to this type of training without any attempt at stress management can result in detrimental effects on physical and mental health. It's like driving your car at full speed in second gear all the time. Something , at some point, will give.

So, while this is one approach that is interesting to explore now and then (I will give some suggestions later on) it is by no means the standard Systema mindset.

The standard Systema mindset is what we term "professional." We can think of this in terms of a reasonably good professional in any field, who goes about their work in a non-stressed state, functioning at a cogent and fluid level of ability. Think of actors, pilots, soldiers, musicians, surgeons, paramedics, and so on. Each is able to fully function under the stress of the situation.

This is contrast to the "feral" approach, which tells us that under stress our capabilities degrade to such a level that only

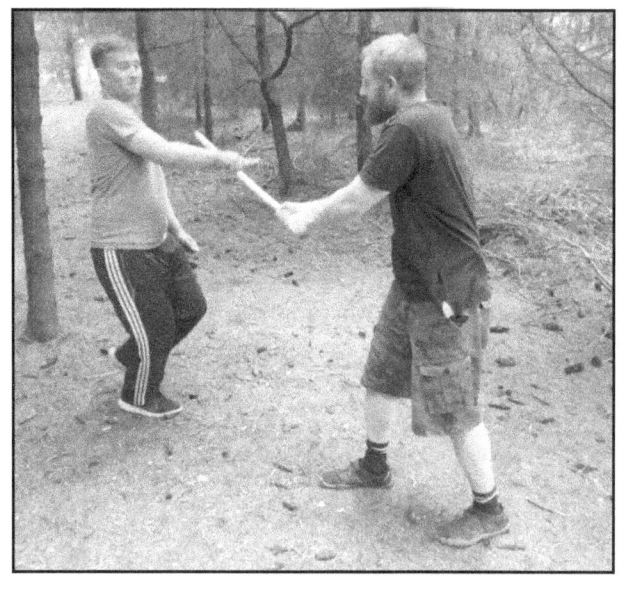

gross motor movement is possible. This is plainly not the case, as the above examples show. Can you imagine a situation more stressful than a heart transplant? Yet a surgeon is able to carry out the minutest and most precise movements during the procedure. A pilot, at high speeds, has a second, if that, to make a decision in an emergency situation. A concert pianist is able to play, from memory, an entire Beethoven piece in front of hundreds of people.

There are countless other examples. "Ah, but," the feral people might say, "fighting is different!" No it isn't. The interesting thing about humans is our fear and reaction mechanisms are the same whatever the stress or perceived threat. Same chemicals, same "butterflies", same potentially overwhelming fear.

Knowing this is one of the keys to training the professional mindset. All we have to do is replicate a situation in order to induce the fear reaction, then bring management mechanisms into play . Again, I will details some ideas for this later on.

For now, it is enough to know that we a re looking, as much as possible, for class training to be carried out in a calm mindset, even in the more challenging drills. The relaxation we spoke about earlier is the bedrock of this, and how you present a class overall will have a major bearing. Depending on the students, you may need to explain or reinforce the concept of "professional mindset" as outlined above. You might even draw on the knowledge of the group, that may be from a professional level or just life experience.

We have had people talk about their work and how they dealt with a particular situation. Another recent example was one of the regulars talking about a car crash he was in a few years back. He hit a fence at speed and one of the fence posts smashed through the window and impaled him under the arm.

He managed to get out of the car and off the road. He lifted up his clothing to examine the wound. It was a cold day and he noticed "breath" coming out of the wound. He removed his top and stuffed it into the hole and clamped down on it to plug the wound. He then lay on the side of the wound on the verge, in order to put more pressure on it. Fortunately a passing car pulled over and called an ambulance.

In hospital it was found out that our friend had a punctured lung (hence the "steam") and had several broken ribs. The staff thought he had been thrown out of the car, and were quite surprised when he told them "No, I got out and walked away."

Later on, when speaking about this in class, he recounted how his mind was very clear and calm, he was focused entirely on what he had to do. There was no panic, no "feral" behaviour though, of course, shock set in later on! A remarkable story, yet in some ways not that remarkable given the capabilities of humans when they allow themselves to operate under stress rather than being shut down. I'm sure anyone you know who works in the emergency services will tell you of many similar incidents.

FLOW STATE

This professional mindset is also an aspect of what has come to be known as flow state, or *being in the zone*. It is a state that all of us have experienced at some time or another. It might be through being totally engrossed in a book. It might be as we take the prefect shot in golf, or get lost while playing a piece of music.

The term first came about through the work of psychologists Mihaly Csikszentmihalyi and Jeanne Nakamura, and describes a feeling where, under the right conditions, you become fully immersed in whatever you are doing. "There's this focus that, once it becomes intense, leads to a sense of ecstasy, a sense of clarity: you know exactly what you want to do from one moment to the other; you get immediate feedback," Csikszentmihalyi said in a 2004 TED Talk.

I cover flow state in more detail in *Systema Self Defence*, but here's a very quick and easy drill you can run in order to get people into it. This is something we often do near the start of a session, or at the beginning of our longer workshops and camps.

We need a group of around six people. One, the catcher, stands on a spot. The others, the throwers, arrange themselves in a semi-circle in front of the catcher. We begin with one stick. The stick is thrown (sensibly) to the catcher, who immediately returns it to any of the throwers, who then throws it back to the catcher.. One function of this drill is to improve awareness and peripheral vision from the catcher. If the stick is dropped, one of the throwers picks it up, the catcher does not move from their spot. Once the catcher has settled in, introduce another stick. So now the catcher has to track two sticks. Increase to three or four as required.

We find that the level of focus required in this drill very quickly brings people into a flow state. They have no notion of time, the task requires attention but is not too challenging, there is no time to think, just to act. In fact, Ed Philips told me a story this morning about this.

He had a new student to class and was explaining the professional mindset and acting without thought. The new student said to him "but it's impossible to not think." So he got the group to run through the stick catch drill. The new student was up to catching and throwing three sticks, when Ed asked her, "what are you thinking about?" to which she replied, "nothing, really." Job done!

As with our relaxation it is one thing to explain flow state, we can even show diagrams and talk about the Nine Requirements of Flow (see Appendices). Or we can throw and catch some sticks! Once people experience that state, once they have that internal connection, they will understand what you mean and, furthermore, will be able to access that state more readily in the future.

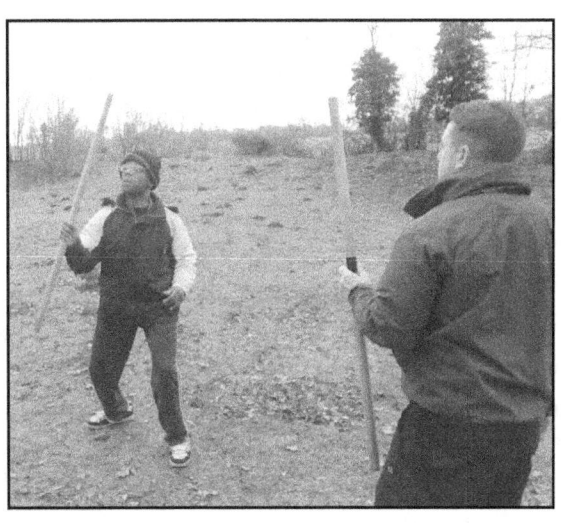

So this type of drill is one of the best in the toolbox - in fact, I'd even venture to say that the majority if Systema drills are designed to put us into flow state - because that is the exact mindset we hope to be in during any type of stressful situation.

Naturally, this does not mean that we can just throw a few sticks around then expect to act like James Bond if someone pulls a gun on us. Same as with the breathing, same as with the relaxation, we have to learn how to access those skills or that state under different types of pressure. However the important thing is that, unlike the "just go feral" approach, we are giving people the tools to counter the stress and adrenaline, so allowing them to access the required skills and attributes.

One last thing to mention on this subject. I spoke earlier about the concept of degradation to basic movements under pressure, how some view it as impossible to do any kind of refined movement. Well, when we think of typical Systema movements, what are they? Quite natural movements, up, down, side to side, figure eight and so on. Nothing complex, nothing that requires memorising fixed patterns. This means that students can hit the ground running as far as self defence goes. They can pick up a measure of ability very quickly as they already have the tools to hand - they just might need a bit of reminding!

This contrasts with those arts that require us to train specific positions or sequences of movements that must then be practiced thousands of times in order to stick in our "muscle memory."

Systema takes the approach that we already have muscle memory. Throw someone a ball, what do they do? Did they train a ball catching kata? No, it is a natural reaction. This is not to say that our reactions cannot be turned into responses, then further refined form more efficiency and effectiveness. But at their root, these are natural, human movements that we perform everyday. Life is our kata, the world is our gym.

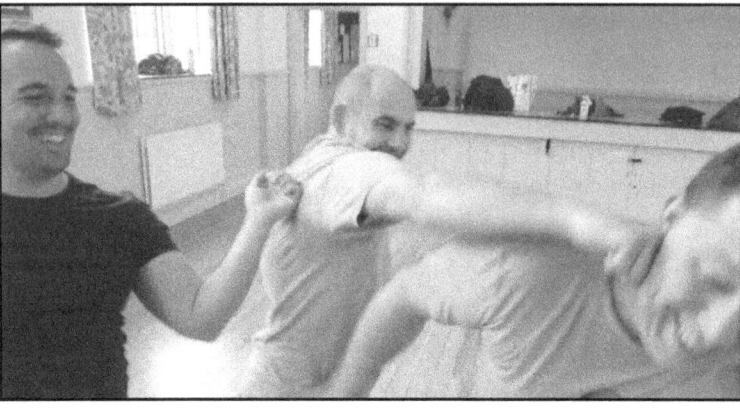

CHALLENGES

Vladimir once said to me, "when you teach, you are on a knife edge," and I knew exactly what he meant. Anything can happen at any time! I imagine there are few teachers in any subject who have not been challenged at some time. The thing is, in martial arts, that challenge is invariably physical!

I've already spoken about the challenge you may get to your teaching. But how do we deal with the more obvious or overt challenge? To the "I don't think that would work," or similar? This can come from inside the group or outside, let's look at the former first.

It is perfectly natural in any student/teacher relationship for there to come a moment where the student challenges the teacher in some way. In much the same way, a child, usually at the teenage stage, will challenge their parents. I'm always reminded of a saying I once heard, "When I was eight, my dad was Superman, when I was 18 he was an idiot, now I'm 48 he's a cool geezer."

As children we believe our parents know everything. Then we find out they don't. Then, particularly when we have kids of our own, we find out, actually they knew a fair bit!

A similar process can go on in a long term teaching relationship, particularly if the student is young. I found this was especially the case in the more traditional Oriental martial arts schools, where the teacher is almost literally seen as the "father."

Now, this challenge may be quite playful, the odd sneak attack here and there. This is actually a healthy thing in the right circumstances. When I trained with Vladimir at his first UK visit, I remember him playfully sweeping a foot as you walked past him. Okay, I thought, two can play at that game. Later on, as he walked past, I swept his foot.

Of course, he effortlessly avoided the sweep and walked on, laughing. This was a very new experience for me, and has always been an aspect of Systema that I enjoy - the playfulness. More on that later.

The next type of challenge may not be so playful. The student wants to test the teacher out, to see if this stuff really works. That may be at different degrees of intensity, and can be problematic. It can also manifest in different ways. I've encountered it most often where you are running through or demonstrating a drill and you get a sudden surge of resistance. I call this "asking a question." But first, let's talk about demos, as it is another important point and relates in many ways to this topic.

Why do we demonstrate? You need to be very clear of this, and it may be a different reason each time. Usually, I am demonstrating in order to illustrate a particular concept, movement, or technique, for the benefit of the group - particularly our "visual" friends! How, then, should a student react to my movements? Should they offer no resistance at all and collapse at my touch? Or should they go all out to prevent what I am doing? The answer usually lies somewhere in-between.

First, we need to have the correct conditions for the drill. In other words, if I am showing a wrist-lock, don't tuck your hands in your pockets.

Second, let the group first see how the technique works. In the above example, I show where I place my hands, the angle of movement, how much pressure to apply and so on.

Third, I may show some variations. At this stage, I am not expecting overt resistance from my partner, they are being quite passive. Not totally, however, because if my angles are wrong, the technique should not work.

Once we are beyond that stage, we can get into the "what ifs." Know my partner my try some escape, or to tense their arm, etc and I can begin to say, "if they react in this why, try doing this." That may be on a technique base, or more of a structure / feel basis. Finally, I can demo how it works in more of a live situation, now my partner can respond more naturally.

There is nothing wrong with explaining this process as you go along. And you can skip levels depending on the experience of the group, it may be you can go straight to the live part. Good students will naturally pick up on where and what is going on, but you may need to explain this process to newer people.

Let's think back to our relaxation section, too. One question is "why should I relax?" I recently saw on of those Youtube clips where a guy calling himself The Strangler or something was criticising Mikhail.

According to this guy, Mikhail was "telling his partner to relax so that his technique will work." So think about what stage of demo we are at. Is Mikhail showing something to teach the basics? Excessive resistance may mean having to change to something else, maybe not the thing that Mikhail wanted to show.

However, also think back to our "both sides benefit" concept from earlier. It may be that one aim of the drill is to help the student relax under pressure.

Far more likely, is that applying the wrong type of tension and resistance to a movement will result in injury to the student, something any instructor would wish to avoid. This goes back to our "asking a question" notion. To me, encountering unexpected resistance in such a case is the person asking "does this really work?" So how do we answer?

It depends very much on the situation. Let's take that wrist-lock example again, as it is a clear one. I take the hand and position for the lock. As I apply it, I feel a lot of tension come up the arm, attempting to lock the wrist in place. One option is to snap the lock on hard and fast. This will do the job, but will most likely injure or even break the wrist.

Another option is to give the arm a tug, in order to extend it out and so break the tension, and then apply the lock safely.

Or, I could relax the arm by giving the person a sharp kick to the shin, then apply the lock. Finally, I could ask the person to relax a little as I don't want to hurt them.

The last time this happened to me was when teaching a group of mostly dancers. We were working a simple takedown from the head and everyone was fine, they got the point of the drill. All except for one chap, who insisted "try it on me, try it on me."

As I placed my hand on his forehead I felt his shoulders and neck fully tense in preparation to resist my movement. So instead of doing the gentle roll I had been demonstrating, I made a sharp movement that resulted in a very loud click from his neck and him dropping like a stone. It was worrying for a second and brought an "oooh!" From the crowd. He was okay, he

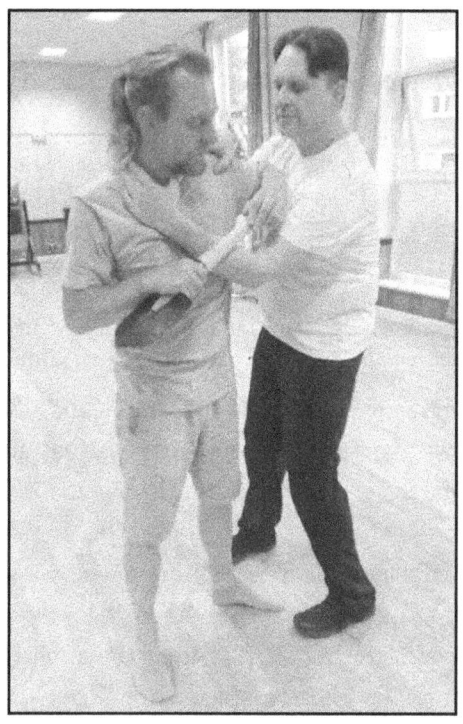

stood up nodding and wandered off, presumably happy - at least, he never asked again! It does illustrate how this can be a lose-lose situation. Fail in your movement and people lose confidence in your abilities. Apply your skills a little more realistically and it might make people uncomfortable.

Generally speaking, I've found that people are smart enough to understand what is going on. If not, and if they keep doing the same thing, the easiest thing is never to use them for a demo! It might be a bit of a cop out, on the other hand, why give yourself the pressure? You will find most instructors are selective with demo partners, especially in a workshop setting where they may not know everyone. This is partly to avoid the problem of being put in that position when you are attempting to teach.

Another aspect of this is the "Oh but I could have..." I heard this recently where someone claimed "yeah, what the teacher was doing to me there, I could have countered it, but I didn't want to embarrass him." Well, it's nice that you are so sensitive to the teacher's feelings, but at the same time you have to wonder what level the teacher was operating at.

By that I mean that generally, in demo mode, an instructor is usually only in first or second gear, and is normally showing something specific for the purposes of teaching. Naturally, as you know what is happening and what they are going to do, you may have a chance to counter it. But why would you, in that situation? Regardless even of that, if you want to ask the question, then be sure that you are prepared for the answer.

As an instructor, I always give students ample opportunity to ask anything, try anything and question anything. However you still occasionally get situations such as the one above, or people like the chap who came to one of my workshops, stood with arms folded most of the time and only lightly engaged, yet afterwards reportedly said something along the lines of "it was all crap, I could've," etc etc. It's not worth worrying over.

The cheap shot is another form of challenge and one that can pop up during demos. In this, the person suddenly goes outside of the parameters of the drill and tries to catch you out. Not especially useful if the instructor is trying to teach something, and potentially dangerous if we are forced to respond quickly. Again it is something of a lose/lose. Fail to react and you get hit. React in "real time" and you may hurt the student.

I heard of an instance of this with knife defence. The student suddenly upped the game in order to test the instructor and ended up with a badly injured arm. As a result, that person never came back, neither did their friends, nor the people who had dropped in to watch the class on that occasion.

It is odd, isn't it? I have heard similar examples from colleagues. A person tests, you deal with it but they get hurt, and they never come back. It makes no sense when you think about it. The challenge was met and dealt with, but you don't want to train there?!?

These are all situations of people from within the class or group being the challenger. What if we have to face an external challenge? In other words, a person comes into the room specifically to fight or challenge you in some way? I don't think it is so commonplace these days these days, maybe times have changed. But back in the "old days" it was by no means uncommon.

From a traditional perspective, it used to be the case that in some styles, a teacher setting up a new class was under an obligation to accept every challenge that came through the door for a period of three months. Following that, if the school was still open, the teacher had the option to refuse, and/or to pass the challenge on to a senior student. I suppose the idea was to ensure that any school opening was genuine, and not some fake or chancer.

What form these challenges took was usually some sort of duel-type situation,

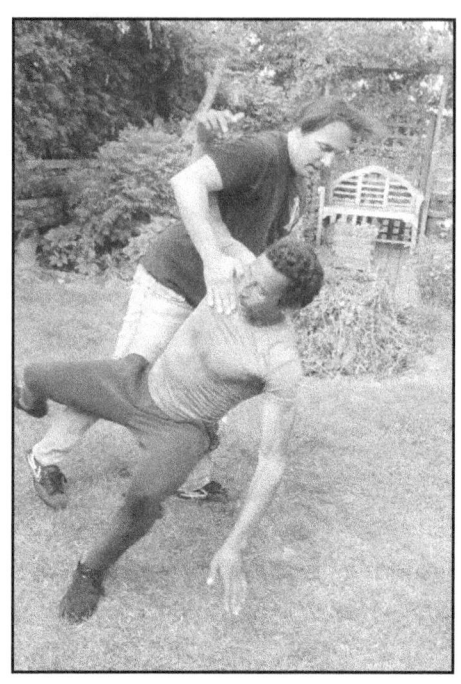

to an agreed set of rules. That may be a polite "cross hands" or a knock-down fight. This was pre-internet, though footage is still around of some challenges, and they used to be a major subject of letter column "flame wars" in martial art magazines.

Being involved in such a situation calls for good judgment and quick decision making. A veteran Karate sensei who was teaching in a rough area told me about a visit he had once from some lads, who he recognised as being part of the local criminal firm. One fronted him out, telling him "karate is useless." Had he backed down he would have lost the class, or perhaps been only allowed to run it under their terms. I asked him what he did, he replied with a smile, "I picked up a chair and knocked him out with it. Never had any trouble after that." Quick thinking, a cool head, but also the knowledge that the particular course of action was the right thing to do. After that he was respected by the gang and went unmolested.

I'm not advising that's what you should do that every time, by the way, just giving an example of how things can go! These days you need to be very wary of any such challenge. You are perfectly within your rights to refuse to engage. Make it clear you have no interest - but do so in a firm, measured way. Don't show fear, don't be aggressive.

Again, in the old days, it was usual for any challenger to be passed on to the senior student. That was part of the job of being a senior, you were expected to uphold the good name of the school. Sometimes senior students would be pitted against each other.

I can think of a few times from those days where challengers would turn up unannounced. The Chinese term for it was "kick school." I think it died out to some extent with the growth of litigation culture, particularly in the USA. Who wants to get sued for throwing a challenger to the floor?

But what do you do if you do get a person or delegation turn up at your class? There's no one answer as there are many variables to consider, which I'll go into in a moment. But if you do decide to go ahead, there are two things that are vital to have in place.

The first is to insist on a waiver. Something of the lines of "both parties accept the course of action may result in serious injury. Neither party will hold the other responsible for any such injuries and will not prosecute or litigate." That is a very rough version, you may even want to get someone with legal experience to draft something for you.

This waiver may be written and signed, or it may be agreed to on camera, which brings us to our second point. These days, it is easy to film anything. Everyone has a phone, I tend to always have a camcorder at class, mostly in order to film sections of the training. However, should there be an incident, be sure that it is filmed.

I would also advise that the encounter be in front of other people. I was involved in an incident some years back where the two of us went into a back room at a

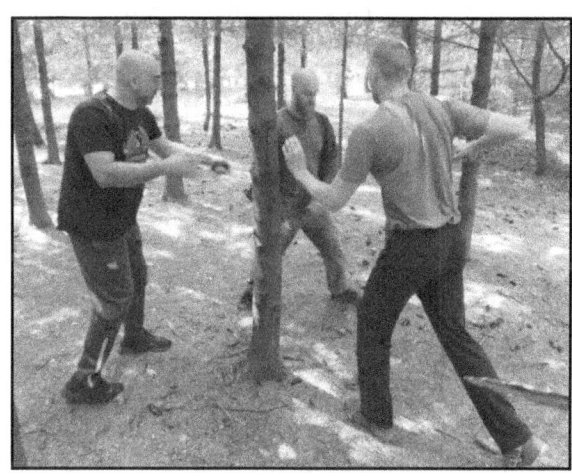

workshop, no witnesses, no cameras. That person's version of what happened changed and grew with each subsequent telling, now I am not even sure that I wasn't actually killed on that day. Problem is, it's one person's word against another, so now I would always make sure there are witnesses and filming.

Before you start, be very clear what the boundaries are. I already mentioned the British Kickboxing rules guy. I don't even know what they are! And surely, if you want to test Systema, then let me do Systema! Another challenger (though reasonable friendly) refused to fight without any mats down. The funniest was the guy who, partway into the challenge, asked me to "stop moving around so much so I can hit you."

You should at least agree if there will be any gloves or protective gear, is this grappling only, levels of contact and so on. Then you have to watch out for the cheap shot, of course, especially if the other person starts struggling.

You should also be prepared to lose. You aren't the best in the world, no-one is. Anyone can get caught out. Generally speaking, especially if the other person had a decent attitude, I took these incidents as a learning experience. In fact, one of my best friendships came about through one. It was when I was teaching Chinese arts, and a guy called Rob Murray turned up.

Very capable fighter, but a nice guy. He asked if we could "spar around" after class and I agreed. I can still remember how he lifted me above his head and put me gently down on the floor!

It was a little like my first encounter with Vlad - done with honesty and respect, no attempt to dominate. I spent many years training with Rob at his home gym in North London, we used to exchange a lot of information and try out all types of things. Good days.

I mentioned variables, so let's examine a few of those. The first thing you should determine is the mental state of your challenger. Once or twice I've had people with obvious issues coming into class. You should handle these people with as much care and compassion as possible. We had one guy in who was clearly drunk. Again, no need to engage, you should be able to handle this verbally.

If a person is being extremely aggressive and you feel a real threat, you always have the option of calling the police. At the very least, try to get them off the premises - and make sure they are not hanging around outside afterwards. It may well go against the grain, you may find yourself gritting your teeth, or worrying that you are in some way chickening out in front of your students. To be honest, if they are not mature enough to grasp the reality of such a situation, they may not be the people you want to each.

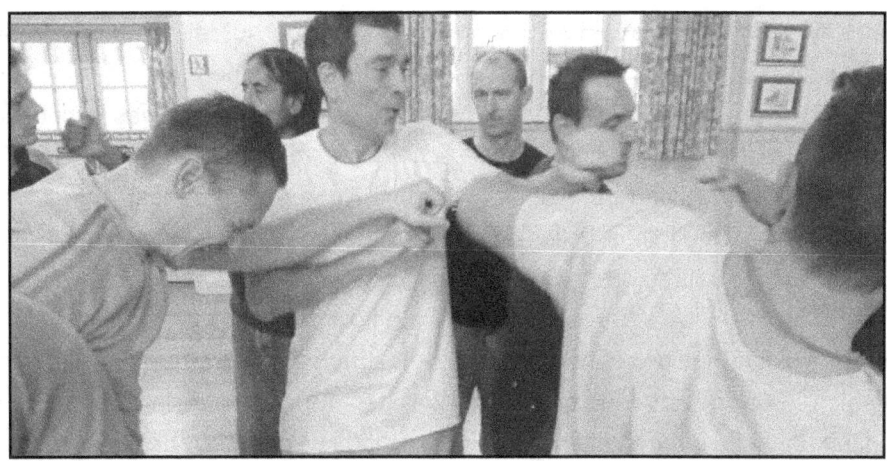

If you do have to engage, first make it verbally very clear (for the benefit of the camera) that you are acting purely in self defence and have no wish to hurt your attacker.

After that, be quick and decisive, don't play around. Do your best not to harm or injure your attacker, but not at the expanse of your own safety. With a reasonable skill level, you should be well equipped to deal with an average person, both physically and psychologically. Against a skilled person, well, it comes down to relative abilities and luck.

Speaking of psychology, don't neglect this area. A Kung-fu instructor I knew always had a gum shield in his pocket. He used to get a number of people coming in off the street for a challenge. He would put the gum shield straight in and say "Okay, let's go!" The challenger backed down every single time.

In short, think this scenario out and come up with a few strategies. You might even want to run through them with your group, make it a drill. Explore all the different ways to deal with the situation, much the same as we do with a robbery, road rage, etc.

You may find that you have students willing to step up for you, and this is fine, too. I've never done this, but I have used a good student in another way. Sometimes you might get a difficult person in, the sort of person who never challenges the teacher, but starts going heavy on fellow students. Sometimes this can be through fear or inexperience, and is rectified with a little chat. Other times, it is bullying or ego. So once or twice I've teamed such a person with one of the experienced guys and given them the go ahead to "give as good as you get." I found that the person either never returns or, even better, adjusts their attitude accordingly and modifies their behaviour.

One last incident, which relates back to the student challenge, but was done in a "positive" way - at least that's what the student thought! I was called in to teach self defence to a group of office workers in Cambridge. At the first session, we started with a little chat, then I explained that I'd show some of the things we would be covering over the course. In my mind, this meant some simple breakaway techniques, avoiding being grabbed, that kind of thing. To the student that I'd brought along to help, it meant launching a full-out assault, he came in shouting, flailing wildly, like a berserker! I had to drop him on the spot with a fast takedown, crashing him to the floor.

The group of nice office people stood aghast. Only three came back next week. I asked the student afterwards what he was doing, his reply was, "I wanted to make it look realistic, you know, make it look good."

So he was coming from a well-intentioned place, but with a complete misunderstanding of the requirements of the situation. A good lesson on my part on not taking things for granted and explaining prior to any such demo in the future!

EMOTIONS

Something else I have found with Systema in regard to other arts, is that it fully explores the are of human psychology and emotion. In virtually all other arts I have studied, emotion was ignored, repressed even, in favour of either that "predator mindset" I mentioned before, or a sort of pseudo-calm that I think was supposed to echo someone like Kwai-Chang Cain from the old *Kung Fu* TV series (in fact I even remember one guy who very much adopted the speech patterns of the main character!)

So how best to approach this subject as an instructor? There are two things to consider, emotions arising naturally, and drills that are specifically designed to prompt an emotional response.

Consider even our "simple" selective tension exercise mentioned earlier. We know that emotional stress is manifested and stored in the muscles. Therefore, even releasing tension in the muscles can release corresponding emotions. This may be a "quiet" process for many, people simply feel the negative emotion "sliding away." However, it can also prompt a more overt response, such as crying or laughter.

This is something you should talk about in class at some point, again with the caveat of context. If you were running an Control & Restraint course for security staff, for example, I wouldn't expect this to be a major concern. However, should those people wish to delve deeper in future sessions, that is another kettle of fish. I also wouldn't necessarily belabour the point with new students, either, give them a chance to settle in. Having said that, you may spot a person that you feel is particularly stressed on vulnerable, in which case keep an eye on them early on.

How to react if a person has an emotional reaction? We should be supportive but not overly so. Offer the person some comfort, have them sit out to one side, sit and chat with them a bit and so on. Do not make a big deal out of the event though, the last thing you want is everyone gathered around the person asking "Are you okay? Are you okay?" Give the person some time and space to process what is happening to them. When they are ready, they can rejoin the group, or step out of the session if they don't wish to continue.

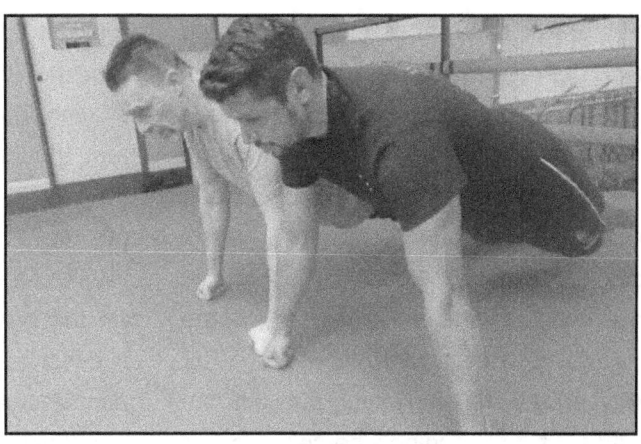

At no point should there be any judgment and certainly no sarcasm or mocking. We can never be sure how other people react to strong emotion - some feel embarrassed or uncomfortable with it. Others may have some experience. In our group we have a couple of students who are also therapists, used to working with people dealing with heavy trauma. If you have access to similar, it is well worth asking for advice and/or help should the need arise. I might also team that therapist up with a student I think may be approaching that point. This is something you learn to pick up on with experience.

We should also mention neuro-diversity and mental health issues here as well. It can be a difficult area, as a person's emotional or mental state is not always readily apparent. Prior to Systema, I had a couple of students experiencing mental issues. Back then, there was far less awareness of such issues, and it was challenging, particularly when the situation escalated to unannounced home visits. Fortunately, I had some good guidance from a friend, and both situations were positively resolved.

These were rare incidents in decades of teaching, but it is something to be aware. Fortunately, attitudes have changed considerably and there is much more guidance and support available. Of course, you can also talk directly to the person, or to a partner or parent. Currently I've had one young man attend class with his mother, she explained his issues beforehand and, knowing that in advance, we have been able to fit him in very nicely with the rest of the group.

Another emotion that may surface during training is aggression. This is often based in fear, in fact I would say almost always so. If you are monitoring the class, you should be aware of the signs. We have already spoken about over-competitiveness, however there may also be a flash of temper. A person my be triggered by being hit on the site of an injury, or by being emotionally put back into a bad situation. Imagine a person who had undergone violent assault suddenly being grabbed and pinned to the floor in class, for example.

Communication is key again, making it clear that all work is consensual and conducted within strict guidelines. A triggered response may be down to a partner going out of those guidelines, or it may cause the responder to go outside. Either way, the situation needs to be dealt with quickly. Separate the people involved and give them time and space to consider what happened. If you are okay with them rejoining the class, best to keep them apart for the rest of the session, maybe even into the future.

This can prove a challenge, but we have to recognise that sometimes people just don't get on! I had two students who, apart, were as good as gold. Whenever they paired up though, there was some sort of flair up. It never really got physical but voices were raised and it was clear they had issues with each other. I got around it by simply never pairing them up and, after a chat and a short time, the situation improved. I still keep an eye on them, though!

Let's move on to drills that are designed to provoke an emotional response. We begin with the breathing /selective tension work as described. This gives the student an opportunity to experience this type of work at their own place. Many may be unfamiliar with this approach, particularly if they come from more "external" martial arts, or the type of background the encourages the repression of emotion, particularly in men.

The second stage is to work with a person. This initially takes place of helping them to relax through manipulation of their structure, using throws and ground work and taking strikes. Of course, the work should all be progressive, starting at a level of reasonable comfort and gradually increasing in intensity.

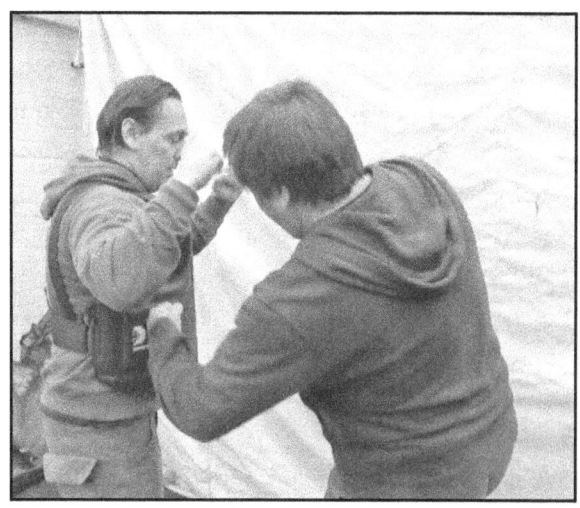

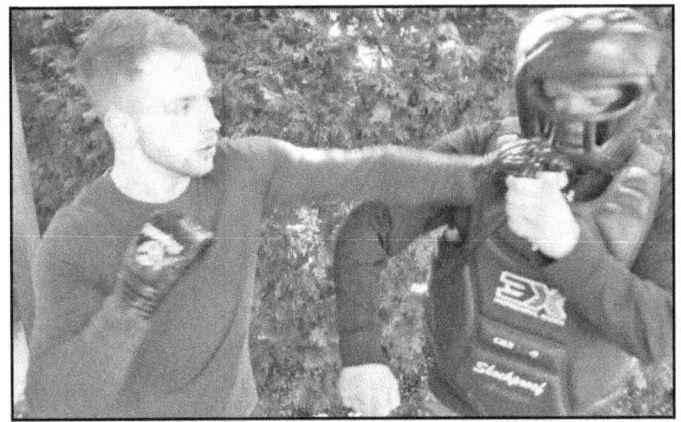

At some point, though we have to go beyond a comfort level in order to access the student's inner state. This is often referred to as "cracking the egg without harming the check."

Over time, we all build up "armour." This is where the body develops ,muscular tension in order to either shield itself from outside threat, to to bury within feelings of trauma or distress. A simple example would be to imagine you once badly damaged your knee. That knee is perfectly fine now, fully recovered, yet any quick movement by a person towards that knee will likely result in a flinch on your part. The knee naturally moves away. This is one aspect of the body's shielding mechanism.

On a deeper level, let's imagine that a person underwent some form of bullying as a child. It may not have been physical violence, maybe it was purely verbal. This may lead to a situation where the sound of a raised voice, or any type of visual or verbal aggression again causes that flinch reaction, even to the extent of the person shutting down.

Neither situation is ideal and needs to be addressed. That is on purely a practical "self defence" level. But we think beyond that, too. Allowing past experiences to influence, even control, or current and future selves, is not a recipe for a happy life. At some point we need to "let go" and move on.

Drills to achieve this mainly involve placing the student under great and greater degrees of stress and tension, "cracking" the shield and allowing the repressed emotions to escape. You generally find that once they are gone, they are gone. Of course, the deeper the trauma, the more work may be needed.

And this is on-going work, too, because we a subject to stress and tension every day of our lives. But the genius of Systema is that under-going this process not only releases stuck emotions but also teaches us how to manage our stress-response in the future. Far better to not let he stress penetrate in the first place, or, if it does, to be bale to neutralise it immediately.

This process can be remarkably simple - just hit people! How we hit as important, and much of this is written about in Vladimir's excellent *Strikes* book. But here's a starting guide to beginning this process. Let's say we have a new student, after a few lessons we can begin the strikes work.

First, explain what is going to happen and the purpose of the drill. No need to go too much into details, just explain we are learning how to take strikes, how to manage impact, how to deal with fear and the tension it brings. The student should also have a reasonable grasp of breath work, particularly burst breathing.

Stand to one side of the student and show them your fist, simply position it a foot or so away from their abdomen. If they flinch or tense, get them to go into burst breathing and release the tension. Repeat as necessary.

Now do the same but move the fist closer. Finally work with contact. Just place your fist onto the student's abdomen. Follow the same procedure, allow the student to breath away any tension.

Next, place the fist and lightly push in. Just enough to move the student or break their structure a little. Emphasise the importance of breathing - as the push comes in, they should exhale, to the same speed and depth. Physically, there are some different methods to deal with a strike, at first I recommend this - you have the student relax in order to absorb the push. Show them how the hip can roll back to neutralise the movement, for example. Be sure to mention the importance of maintaining form and posture as much as possible, but without being overly tense.

From there, progress to an actual strike. Light at first, just at skin level. Be sure not to hit the same spot over and over and try not to work to a rhythm. At any sign of undue discomfort or distress, drop back a level. From light hits to pushes. From pushes to touch, etc..

Over time, increase the depth and power of the hits. Always give the person time to recover between hits. At some point, you need to put just enough in to wind the person and force them into burst breathing. You should also vary the location, especially to the face. When you switch, you can also go back down the scale, starting with light contact again.

If you are working specifically to trigger emotion, then a slap to the face will usually do the job. Exercises your judgement as to how heavy this should be - you may find that just a light tap can elicit a strong response.

Another word on this work - be very sure that you are never presenting it in egotistical terms. Always be aware that a person is standing you still and letting you hit them. You may think you have a powerful strike after doing this, but this is not a live situation. Also, never use this work in order to establish your dominance, unless absolutely necessary. I had word from a friend who attended a class of one instructor who, at

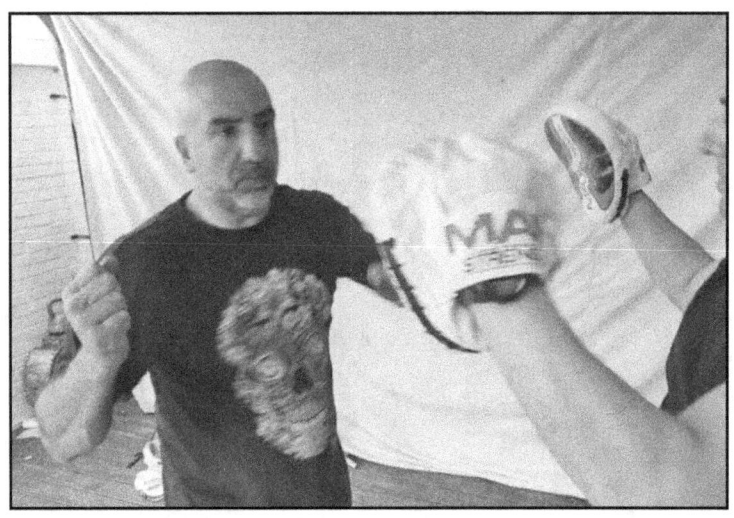

the start of the session, would line all the students up then go along belting them hard in the guts. This is the sign of an insecure instructor. We are here to teach, not to bully, beside which all he was doing, in most cases, was reinforcing fear, not helping people overcome it.

When you feel a student is ready, you can move on to the next level. I'll describe my personal experience of this, and you can take from it what you will. I think it was my third visit to Toronto, and I had my wife with me. Towards the end of my visit, it may have even been my last class, Vladimir called me forward and, for what felt like ten minutes, basically beasted me round the room. I was told I could move and try to escape, some hope! I was punched, kicked, thrown, it was all I could do to keep breathing and moving.

I'd add that his strikes were not injurious, but they were deep. Vladimir exercises perfect control. In fact, I even had the imprint of his foot on my shoulder after! As far as I remember, the rest of the group were watching. At the end of the beating Vladimir sat me down and gave me a sort of massage around my head and shoulders, it was a reassuring feeling and did something to bring my back into myself. He left me to sit quietly for a while and the class resumed. Afterwards, I said my goodbyes and off we went.

We were spending another day in town visiting relations, and the next morning I was in the bath in our hotel room. I had the most peculiar feeling of something inside me opening up and letting go. It felt like years of tension and fear came flooding out, the deepest emotional release I have ever experienced. That night, and for a few nights after, I slept like a baby. And during the day my entire body felt unusually light, it was the closest I can think of , without being over-dramatic, to a feeling of being "re-born."

It was at that time I began to realise, understand and appreciate something of the true depth of Systema and its capacity for very quick, deep and, above all, positive

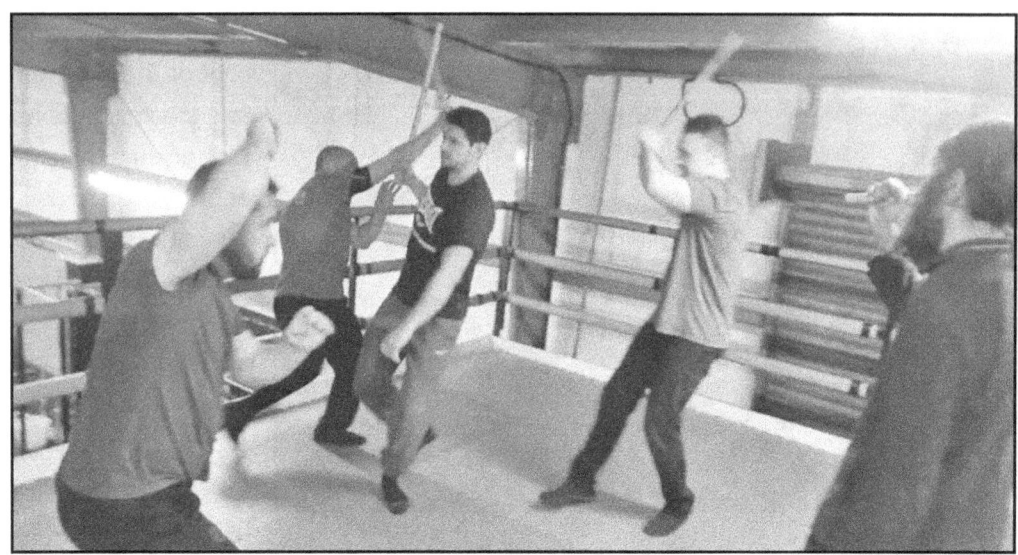

transformation. You may have had similar experiences and thoughts too, and that this is an aspect of Systema you wish to share with others. That is laudable, but, as I mentioned before, take your time and be sure you are not "forcing the medicine" on anyone. Present your work calmly and professionally, and people will come to you for this kind of work.

How you do this yourself will vary. My first attempt was basically to try and replicate what Vladimir did to me. It was okay-Ish, but with time and practice I learnt how to be more subtle in the work, how to assess the individual and adjust accordingly. I don't think this is a skill than can be directly taught - you have to first under-go the experience and then gradually develop your own approach to applying it.

In fact, we have come up with some variations on the drill. This is useful as not everyone wants to undergo the "beasting" experience. However, we have found using things like stress positions, blindfolds, and so on have been useful - again all with the big caveat of responsible use!

RELATIONSHIPS

Wherever we get a group of people, we get relationships. My experience with Systema training has been overwhelmingly positive, in that those who train regularly become a close knit group. This leads to a good atmosphere in class, where people trust each other, which lessens ego and improves the learning experience.

This allows us to explore and emphasise the play aspect of training. When no-one has anything to prove and the group is "in synch", the training can develop in many interesting ways, leading into the deeper aspects of Systema. *Play*, I have come to learn, is not a word that goes down well in martial arts circles. Yet, without fail, this is the primary method of learning to fight amongst humans (and animals!) since the year dot.

The fundamental concept of play is that we seek to prolong the situation in order to learn. This is in contract to a real situation, which we invariably wish to bring to a conclusion in a short a time as possible.

Positive relations, then, lead to better learning. This doesn't mean we are "nice" to each other all the time, the best friends are those who are totally honest with you. They also break down barriers, which can only help with the flow of information. Teachers who are distant, remote figures, who never engage, are not a good source of learning. Likewise, having that good communication means students willing to share expertise and experience, wether in the circle up or during the training.

We've already mentioned how, even with the best will in the world, people don't always get on and how to manage it. But there is one other area of class relationships I'd like to touch upon. A teacher can be seen as a figure of authority. Someone to look up to, to be admired. This can lead to people developing a certain view or even feelings for the instructor. That may be placing the teacher on a pedestal, it may be from a romantic or sexual angle. To be honest, this is not something I've experienced in Systema, though it was not unknown in previous styles.

I think if you are running a decent type of class, there should be little chance of the former happening. None of us are perfect, nor do we present ourselves as such. We should be doing the work and taking the this just as much as the students.

For the second situation, I take the view that as a teacher I am a professional in my workplace, and apply the same approach as if this were a work situation. Having said that, I met my first long-term girlfriend at work, so there is that! However, I personally would not condone the actions of one school that I knew, where any and every student of the opposite sex was seen as "fair game" by the instructor, with attendant innuendo and borderline "grooming."

It behoves us as instructors to present a good example, particularly when it comes to honesty, morality and respecting the

CHAPTER SEVEN
DRILLS & EXERCISES

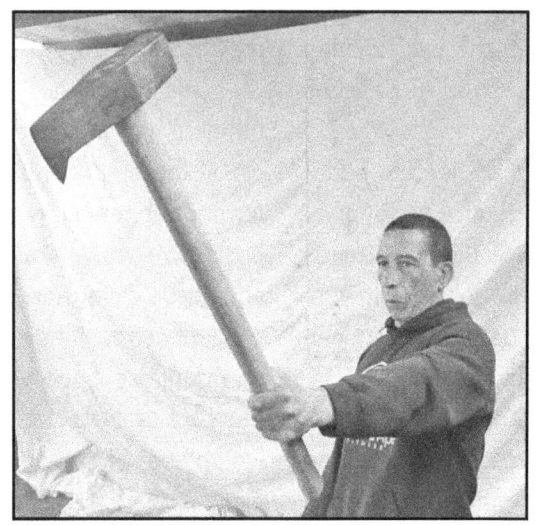

Let's now move on to the actual substance of what we are teaching. I divide this into two categories, exercises and drills. Exercises are those practices designed to develop attributes – mobility, balance, endurance, strength, and so on. They can be practiced solo, in pairs, or in groups.

Drills can be used for attribute training but also cover things like skill acquisition, practical application testing, and so on. Again, these can be solo but are more usually worked in pairs or groups. As mentioned in an earlier chapter, the interesting thing with Systema is that the exercises often map directly onto drills and practical application - a squat is a component of a take-down, and so on.

This means that we can begin the class with exercises that are related to the drills we will be practicing later on, giving the session a nice, cohesive feel. This also reinforces the importance of practicing our exercises away from class, or with the group as described before.

EXERCISES

So we start with the three core movements as our base – push ups, sit ups and squats. We can do these "straight out of the box" or, to add more interest and challenge, we can adapt these exercises in many ways. One method I've found useful, is to adapt through the lens of the Four Pillars – movement, tension/relaxation, breathing and posture. We will take a simple push up as an example.

Standard version – fists under shoulders, spine level, inhale down to the floor, exhale up. Work at the speed of the natural breath.

Movement – think of movement as speed. Work from full speed to as slow as you can and every stage in-between. Also lower down slow, come up fast and vice versa.

Tension/relaxation – as you lower, tense the whole body. As you raise, release the tension. Also work the reverse. Try the whole movement with full tension, then full relaxation. Work with selective tension, eg maintain tension in the legs only.

Breathing – basic in/out with up/down and vice versa. Do three push ups on the inhale, three on the the exhale. Hold the breath for as many push ups as you can. Recover while still doing the push up. Do one very slow push up with burst breathing.

Posture – change position of the hands, feet, legs, etc. Add a sideways roll into the movement. So lower, sideways roll, push-up. Work a push up against the wall, or from an inverse position. Put your feet on a chair, etc.

Already here, then, we have a wide number of variations, not to mention combinations – for example elevated push ups with breath holds. This in itself will give you months of exercise ideas! And this is just solo work, let's add in a partner, too.

I present a wide range of ideas in *Systema Partner Training,* but you can think of your exercise partner in three ways – synchronise, support, resist. Let's continue with our push up example.

Synchronise – partners are shoulder to shoulder and match speed on the push ups. Synch the breathing to help.

Support – one partner holds and elevates the other's feet as they perform the push up. Or one partner lays on the floor and the other does push ups on their body.

Resist – as one partner raise in the push up, the other applies downward pressure to the shoulder, making their partner either push through or work around the resistance.

So another set of simple variations, which we can add to our previous Four Pillar tweaks. Combine these methods, and even with just these three movements we have a very wide range of exercises.

This concept can also be applied to using equipment for exercise. You can synchronise with the stick, by moving it around the body and following its flow. You can use the stick as support by placing its end against a wall and climbing up and down it. You can use the stick for

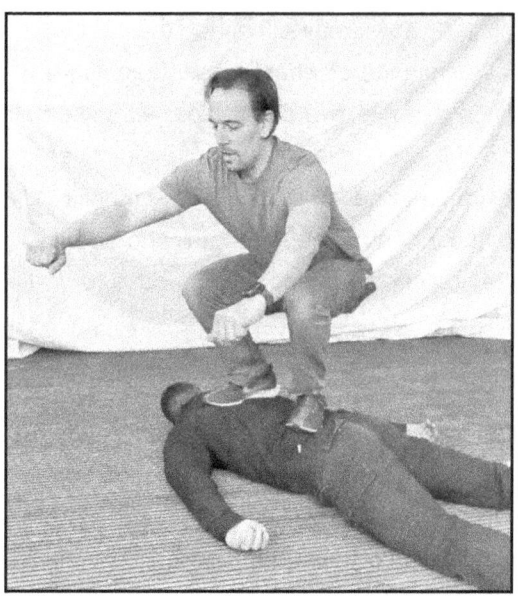

resistance, by twining a leg around it and applying selective tension. The same will also apply to partner work, where your partner is in charge of the stick.

One thing I stress again, is that these seemingly innocuous exercises correlate directly to our practical work - in fact I often refer back to them when we get into drills. Just look at the fist and arm position in a push up and then at a short range punch, for example.

DRILLS

If there are numerous variations for exercises, we can multiply that by ten for drills. The addition of other people into the equation increases variables in countless ways, some expected and some unexpected!

That aside, what differentiates one from the other? To my mind, drills are designed with a specific outcome or outcomes in mind, so let's start there.

When deciding which drills to teach, or when making up your own, the primary consideration is "what is this drill supposed to achieve?" There can be more than one reason, and you may also find students come up with other reasons you didn't think of. But we should begin with a primary reason. Let's look at a series of take-down drills as an example, beginning with how the drill runs.

Stage One: A approaches B, who stands in neutral position. A takes hold of B's arm and moves it slowly out, noting how each position affect's B's structure.

The primary aim at this stage is for A to get a sense of how to manipulate B's posture. For B, the primary aim is to see if they can maintain balance, without offering resistance. In other words, the drill is co-operative.

Stage Two - A now considers the concept of working in three dimensions. We have length, height and width. Show A how to apply this to B's arm. Pulling the arm out forward means altering the length. To the side, the width, and up or down the height.

Pulling the arm one way may result in altering the structure, but adding the second and third dimension will result in B losing balance and falling So have A move the arm in one dimension until they see a change in B's posture. Then repeat, but moving in another dimension. Once the posture is disrupted again, apply the third direction to complete the take down.

At first I would advise applying height last, as this is usually the one that does the trick. The primary aim for A at this stage is leaning to manipulate structure without force or tension, leading to a take-down. The primary aim for B is to recognise when balance is lost and manage the resulting fall and impact with the floor.

Stage Three - A applies their work as above, but now in a more smooth and natural way. Primary aims remain the same but now the work is becoming a little more "real."

Stage Four - B can be more responsive to A, in terms of trying to neutralise the take-down by maintaining structure. The primary aim is now for both to begin understanding structure work in a more dynamic setting.

Stage Five - A and B work against each other. This will be slow at first, building up intensity as required, all the way to full-on grappling. The primary aim now is to apply the previously acquired skills in a live setting. Of course, there are still many restrictions on the drill, as it is not fully live yet, nonetheless those restrictions (eg no strikes, kicks, etc) allow both partner's to fully focus on their grappling skills.

These are the primary goals of the drill but there are others, too. Remind each person of the importance of breathing and monitoring tension levels. You might explain how simple footwork helps with the drill, from both perspectives. You can also add in concepts of wave movement and spirals. Naturally, as the drill progresses we move into areas of head control, collapsing the legs, foot sweeps and so on.

In this way what starts out as a basic "game" evolves into something quite intricate. Hopefully, at some point, you will see both partners drop into that flow state we spoke about earlier. Then you know that the real learning is underway!

THE FOUR PILLARS

We can apply our Four Pillar principles to drills in much the same way as we do to exercises. Of course, all four should be preset in all activities, all the time! But from a teaching perspective it is often useful to slice things down into more digestible chunks.

Most of us, particularly at first, are able to focus on one or two things only when under even the slightest pressure. So let's run through each of the four and suggest some specific drills.

Breathing

A is on the ground, B standing. B walks and A must simply avoid contact. Each partner must maintain a specific breath length, say a four count, as they work. Start slow, with movement matching the breathing. Later, move quicker but with the same length of breath.

Next, add in breath holds on inhale and exhale. Both partners keep moving through recovery / burst breathing stage.

The aim is to first draw attention to breathing, above all else. In this way we allow the body to take over and manage the job of evasion, rather than being too visual and "thinky" about it. This will increase both internal awareness and external sensitivity.

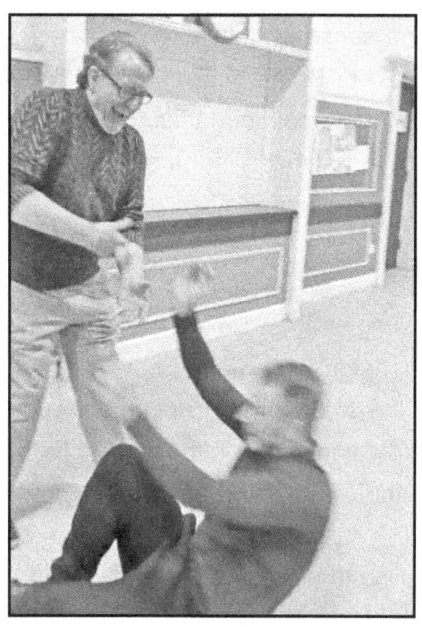

The breath holds function as stress inducers. The challenge is to maintain the same quality of movement while under duress and also to be able to recover on the move. Coordinating breathing between two people, even in a non-cooperative setting, will also increase awareness and lead us into flow state.

Posture
A and B start in clinch position. A's goal is to break B's structure, B's to maintain it. B can use any degree of relaxation or tension (selective) in order to do so. Run the drill for two minutes, then switch the roles. Following that, have both partners work against each other.

The aim is for A to learn how best to break structure through grappling (you can add in strikes later on if you wish). They should pay particular attention to where B's tension is, and their own position and footwork. For B, the aim is to maintain control of their structure under pressure,and, if it alters in some way, to quickly get back into it.

This also teaches the practical use of selective tension, where we can resist without locking the whole body. In the second phase of the drill, we learn how to attack while defending our own structure. Work is primarily by feel, so increasing tactile sensitivity.

Movement
A must negotiate their way through a group of people with minimal contact. Have the group gather in the centre of the room. At first, the group are a little spread out and static. Have people take turns moving from one side or end of the group to the other, with little or no contact.

Each time you cycle round to the first person again, have the group close in a little, until they are in full contact. Following that, have the group spread out again, but this time they are walking around. The group don't impede or interfere with the person moving through, though you can add this in as an option.

The aim is to develop the ability to move smoothly and softly in confined spaces. At first, it is largely training the visual aspect - we see the gap and move into it. You may find it useful to lead with the hand - point the hand into the gap and allow the body to follow.

As the space decreases, we work more from the tactile aspect. When we contact a person, how do we respond? The body should remain soft and slide off / slip around the obstacle. This again reinforces the "feel more than see" principle.

Tension/Relaxation
A stands arm out. The arm is grabbed and B attempt to apply locks. At first A remains neutral. Then A applies full relaxation. Then

A applies full tension to he arm.

Following this, run the same drill but with an extra partner. So now B and C are trying to lock an arm each. A runs through the same procedure. Finally, A applies relaxation to one arm, and tension to the other. The work should be carried out at a steady pace to start, with not too sudden changes of movement. As abilities increase, so can the speed.

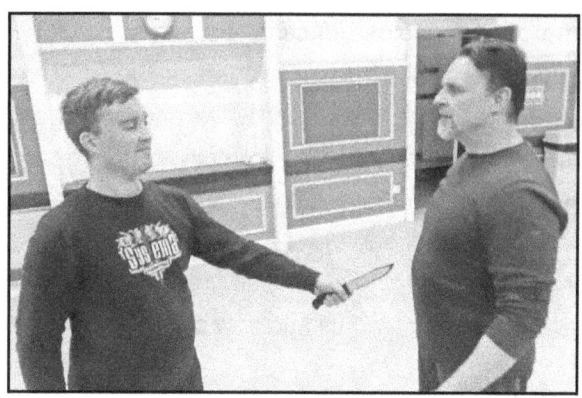

The initial aim is to help A differentiate between varying levels of relaxation and tension while under pressure - which level is more useful in defending against a lock, how to prevent tension from working into the rest of the body and so on. Against two partners, the challenge is to maintain tension against one while being completely relaxed for the other. In other words, this is selective tension applied on the move and against resistance.

It's a useful skill both in muscle control but also in a situation where we may need to hold onto someone tight whilst keeping our other arm free for use against another person.

Four Pillars, then and four drills. No doubt you will be aware of the fact that they all overlap. In the last drill, for example, breaking postures will make it easier for our partner to lock the arm. And, naturally, we are breathing throughout all four! But here is the way this works. In a sense, we sometimes have to fool our students into to doing something that they are not always aware of. In other words, you can present something that looks like an evasion exercises, such as our first example, but actually is focused more on breathing. This hopefully means that while concentrating on breathing, the movement actually improves. Whereas we often find that if you ask people to think only of the movement for that first drill, they don't do as well - too much thinking going on!

So diverting the attention to breathing not only helps with breath control, etc, it also takes away that not very useful over thinking process that ends up actually inhibiting movement rather than enhancing it.

Likewise, in the moving through the crowd drill, if people have done the prior breath work, they will find that although they are concentrating on the movement aspect, the breathing will naturally be smooth and match the situation.

In other words, sometimes it pays to just tell students about one aspect of the drill, and let the others emerge as they will. Astute students will soon pick up on this anyway. It's always nice when you see that realisation dawn on someone's face and they say "Ah, I thought we were doing work against kicks, but this is all about breathing, isn't it?"

It is part of the beauty of Systema that we are able to cover such a wide range of skills in attributes across our training. The difficulty lies in assimilating all of these into coherent drills without over-loading the poor student. "Keep your back straight. Move. No, more smoothly. Inhale, exhale, back straight! Move more. Relax! Relax! Relax!"

How well do you think that works? I remember going to a workshop pre-Systema that had some interesting combatives work, yet the instructor insisted on yelling the whole time like a drill sergeant. In the end I mentioned to him "mate, I don't work any faster or better because you are shouting in my ear."

Now, we all need a bit of encouragement from time to time, but over-loading with information becomes a barrier to learning. So think about this Four Pillar approach and how you can use to to initially focus on just one concept, then gradually bring the others in by stealth.

TIME SLICES

Another way to parse information down is the concept of time slices. With this approach, we focus on one particular moment in time of a situation. Just to widen things out a little first this also relates to my concept of "fighting ranges." Most people categorise these as *kicking, punching and grappling* range (as though you are only bound to do a single on at each range!) I much prefer the time ranges of:
something is going happen, something is happening, something has happened.

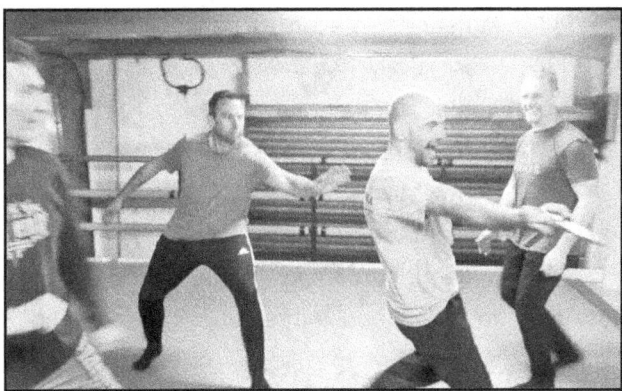

A simple illustration. I'm having a drink in a bar when the guy next to me takes offence at something I said and turns to face me, showing all the signs of aggressive intent. *Something is going to happen.*
Next he reaches out to grab

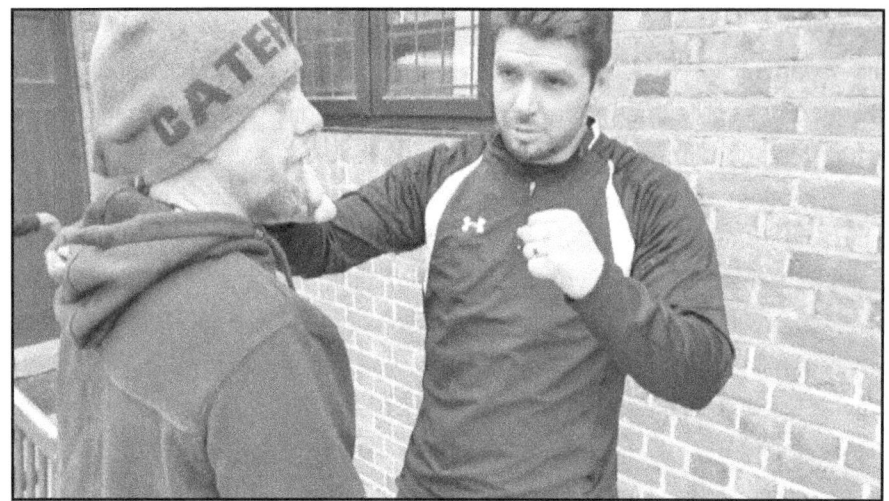

my lapel. *Something is happening.*

Following that, he punches me in the face. *Something has happened.*

Naturally, the earlier we respond in that sequence the better. Or just don't go into dodgy bars! In terms of a drill, this is how we can work that concept.

A the aggressor faces off with B in a belligerent way. B makes a movement, strike or takedown, to neutralise the threat. This is what as known as pre-emptive work, and is legal in most places, as long as you feel under threat and your response is proportionate (check your local laws).

The same set up, this time A moves first into a grab or strike. B makes the appropriate response, neutralising the attack and dealing with the attacker.

And, finally, A now actually grabs or hits B, who has to respond post-contact. In other words, each drill reflects a stage in our sequence.

It is nice to imagine that we always see trouble coming and can avoid it. However, sometimes it may be our job to deal with the trouble, or we may have other people to consider and protect. Still, if we see the trouble coming, we should take the necessary action. However, with the best will in the world, we don't always see it coming. We be already be dealing with one person when their friends intervenes. Or we may be in a crowd, or a dark place, or suffering some form of sensory deprivation - or, surely not, be worse the wear with drink!

Regardless of the reason, we have to know how to respond to that persons movement and also learn to manage impact and contact. So let's go back and refine our earlier three drills into something a little more specific.

Pre-emptive work is largely a function of awareness, and I details an number of good drills in *Systema Awareness*. The first is recognising tension in a person, one of the surest indicators of aggressive intent. A stands opposite B, both in neutral position. B moves a part of their body. On seeing it, A points towards that part area and says "ah!"

Start with very big, clear movements and gradually shrink them down, until B is just slightly tensing a muscle of part of the body. The reason A points and makes a noise, is to get used to the idea of exhale and respond rather than just passively observing.

A stands opposite B, just within touch range. B moves to grab or push A. A must deflect the attacking arm. Think about how this is achieved. If you start slow, it is pretty easy. But as you build up to full speed, it becomes more difficult to catch the attacking arm. This is because A is watching and then reacting to a movement that B has already started. By the time the information goes from eye to brain to hand, the movement is done.

Instead of reacting, B should think of responding. Have B reach for your shoulder to start. Don't react with your hand, but respond by rolling the shoulder back. Use this movement to bring the hand up and it will naturally connect with the attacking arm. Furthermore, the continued roll of the shoulder carries out the deflection part, too.

Think about how people go fishing - they use bait to bring the fish to the hook, they don't go round trying to place the hook in the fish's mouth. Same principle. The attack is drawn in by moving away in the same line. The "hook" is then in place, we can use the hand to deflect, apply our own grab, strike, etc.

Work on this, gradually increasing speed, until you are able to comfortable intercept / deflect grabs to the body. You can then apply the same procedure to punches and kicks.

For the third stage, we allow the grab to...grab. Have your partner apply the grip and explore ways to escape or neutralise it. This might be through movement. For example, if my shirt is grabbed at the front,

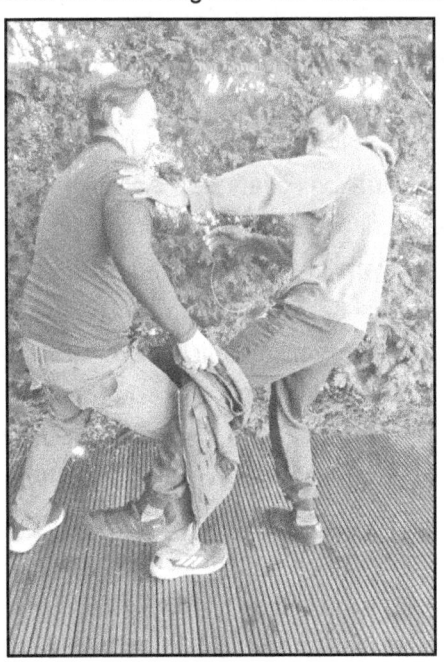

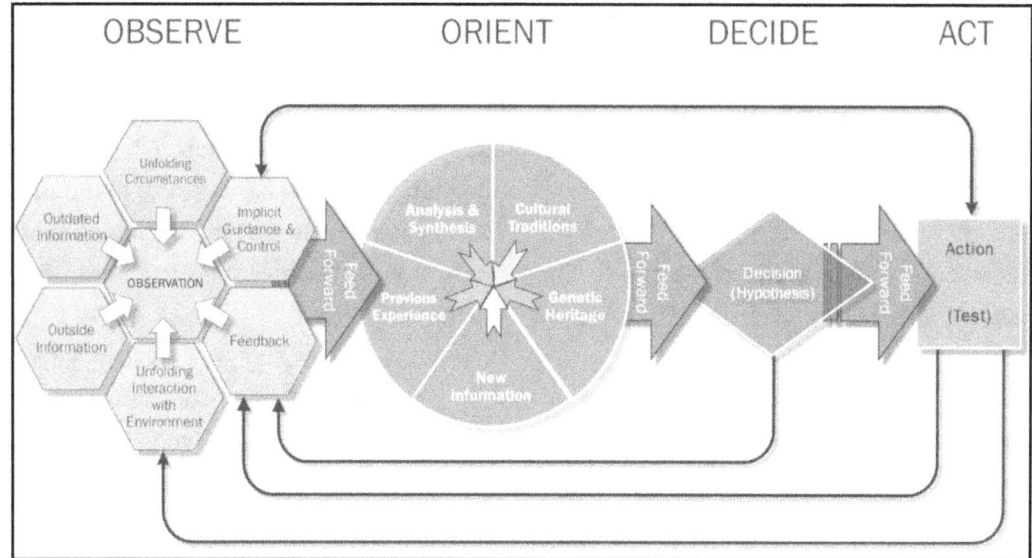

I can usually escape by rolling the shoulder, taking a slight step and twisting the body to the side. Or I may decide to bring my opposite hand over, pin the attacker's wrist to my body, and go into a strike or takedown.

Whichever, I am working from the position of my partner's technique having landed. This is then applied to deeper grabs and holds, punches and kicks. For the latter, be sure to put student's through at least the basics of taking strikes before starting. This will also do a lot to manage any fears of heavier contact.

So there is our first idea of time slicing, but we can go even thinner than that! This also leads us into our area of psychological and non-contact work as, in effect, we are able to work within our attacker's time frame and movements. It also brings us into Colonel John Boyd's OODA Loop territory, again, something I have covered in detail in other books. I'll give a brief description here in case you haven't read those.

OODA stands for Observe, Orient, Decision, Action. Consider this - I Observe the cake tin. I Orient myself by turning towards it. I make a Decision to eat some cake. I make an Action to open the tin and take a slice of cake.

Let's say that somewhere in that process, the situation changes. As I make the Decision, for example, the cake tin moves away from me (horror of horrors!). I know have to re-orient in order to continue. In other words, I drop a step back down the ladder.

Transfer this to an attack. The person Observes and Orients, and is halfway through the Decision making stage when I move away, out of sight. Now they have to start the process again. This is quite a simplification of the process, but nonetheless it works well as an introductory model. It also helps us to begin thinning those time slices down into quite specific sections.

It might also help if you think of them as frames in a movie. We can zoom in to very specific fractions of a second. Speaking of which, when it comes to OODA and the like we are actually dealing with fractions of a second. How fast is a top level tennis serve, around 100 mph? Yet the opposing player sees it and returns it (most of the time!). Why? Because I'd guarantee that their training includes this OODA Loop and time slicing concept.

There is also the phenomena of time distortion, a type of perceptual transformation, sometimes experienced in altered states of consciousness, in which time appears to pass either with great rapidity or with extreme slowness. From our perspective, this is most often associated with the flow state we spoke about earlier, but can also be another effect of understanding the time slice work at a deeper level.

What drills are best to get us into this area of work? Well, we start with the ones already described, the three time ranges. Now take one single part of any of those, and zoom in on it. Let's work with the grab, and look at the actual split second that the grabbing hand first makes contact.

This work needs to be practiced slowly to being with, for obvious reasons. We extend that split second out as long as possible in order to give a chance to formulate a response to it. If we work at full speed from the start, that split second is over in, well, a split second - no chance to learn anything.

So, B reaches slowly for A, to grab the shirt or lapel. A makes no move until the fingers are touching the shirt. As they begin to close, A, matching B's speed, slightly rotates their shoulder back. This, if done correctly, will not quite break contact with B, but will not quite let them fully close the grip either. Furthermore, it should extend B's arm out slightly as they continue to reach for the shirt.

Because they have contact, the brain is fooled into thinking the technique is done. This is why the arm keeps reaching. If the movement is stopped, the brain realises that the move has failed, and resets. In a sense, what we are doing here is not breaking the OODA Loop but keeping it going. We don't want our partner to readjust, we want them to continue with the grab.

Once B's arm is extended out a little, the elbow is vulnerable. It may also lead to B breaking structure and/or losing balance, perhaps with a little help from A.

I hope that example is clear. This is one of fundamental concepts of Systema and one ting that, I believe, sets it apart from anything else I've studied. It's one of the best reasons to do slow training, a method that is so often misunderstood and/or derided by some. Yet it is the same method used by high level professionals in may other activities, and with good reason - because it's effective!

So once your students have a reasonable grasp of the usual grab/punch etc drills, begin to work this time slice concept in. Think of it as almost a masterclass level once people have the basics, or if they have good previous experience in other styles. This is were the work begins to transform from the "normal" A does this, B does that, to the sort of thing we see in good Systema - the improvisation, the seemingly off the cuff response to any type of attack that at once fits naturally and perfectly into an attacker's movement.

THE TEN POINTS OF SPARRING

In *Systema Self Defence* I go into detail on a concept I formulated and titled the Ten Points of Sparring. I'll cover those points here, briefly, as they provide an excellent template for adjusting drills. You can think of the points as a type of graphic equaliser (if you are old enough to remember what one of those is!). Each point can be slid up or down, in endless combinations.

POINT ONE - SPEED
Speed is a simple variable to understand. You can walk very slowly, you can jog, you can sprint. In drill terms it means regulating the speed at which we move, punch, grapple, etc. Usually, we will match speeds for everyone involved in the drill, but occasionally you can mix speeds up for an extra challenge.

Almost every drill starts slow - especially if it is a new drill and new students. Slow sparring is a very useful tool for skill development. Let's assume we are working strikes. We may set the speed at around a quarter of normal speed – so it looks like we are working in slow motion. However, this doesn't mean we work "limp," it is important to maintain the same level of intent as if we working at full speed. This allows us to start reading our partner's body language.

See, for example, how a person lifts the shoulder before throwing a jab. Working at slow speed takes a lot of the fear away, and

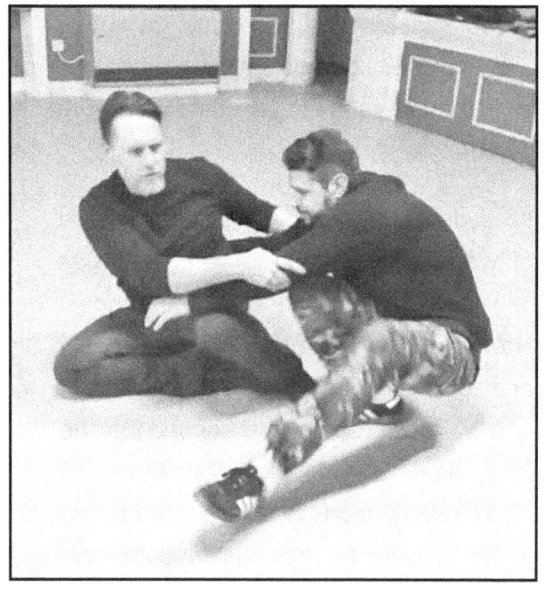

gives us a little thinking time to work out the best response. The same applies both visually and on a tactile level – the brain/body has time to feel and respond to contact. This way we start to develop the ability to take in and process information at a faster rate - because as you increase speed, you will find you are still taking in the same amount of information that you were slowly.

The biggest challenge in working slow is to maintain a constant speed. If fear takes over, or if we see a chance opening, we may suddenly speed up to escape or to hit our partner. This tends to be contagious, as one person speeds up, so does the other. Fear and tension spread very quickly if we are not careful.

The single most effective way to control our speed is through breathing. After all speed tends to be a function of the nervous system, which in turn can be regulated most effectively through the breath.

So prior to any slow work I will normally take the group through some breathing exercises, particularly ladder or square breathing patterns. Have them not only maintain the breath pattern during the drill, but also synch with their partner's breathing, too. This will not only keep the speed even, it will help in achieving flow state.

POINT TWO - DISTANCE

Range is most important factor for any weapon. A good understanding of range is important, along with position, angles and relative distance. Timing is a key concept in fighting and can help overcome many advantages an attacker may have.

Distance is an easy variable to put into place. Generally speaking, the greater the distance the more time we have to react and so the easier things are. When we feel under pressure we tend to try and create more distance between ourselves and our partner. This becomes apparent in some types of sparring, where, even with protective gear, people stay just out of hitting range, then jump in and out with a quick jab or strike.

It is okay to work at this extended range, but there needs to be a good reason for it. One reason is to help people acclimatise to an attack. Working at a distance gives the person a clear visual line of attack and some time to avoid it. This begins to teach angles of attack and the best positions to move to.

On the other hand, we can also start work up very close - for example with a knife actually contacting the body. This helps people get accustomed to the feel of a metal knife and, when the point is pushed into the body, helps develop tactile sensitivity, awareness and reaction against a stab. This may form part of a disarming technique, or it may be damage limitation if a stab does get through to the body. It is also a good drill to promote relaxation of the major muscle groups.

Other drills call for the range to change - the aim may be to learn how to close distance quickly. Distance drills do not necessarily have to be about avoidance, they can also be used for awareness and sensitivity training. For example, the drill may be to remain at a close distance and follow / copy another person's movements. This can be further complicated by having someone simultaneously copy your movements. This type of training is very good for developing reactions, free movement and the ability to "read" and pre-empt someone else's moves.

If we are working to maintain a set distance, we of course primarily work visually. However we can add in tactile elements too. The partners might have a stick or a ball placed between them, which they have to not let fall. You can use a rope or scarf tied to each partner's wrist or ankle in order to stop them moving apart.

POINT THREE - CONTACT

Levels of contact can range from none at all through to landing a strike as hard as you can. The norm tends to be somewhere in between. As a rule we prefer to always

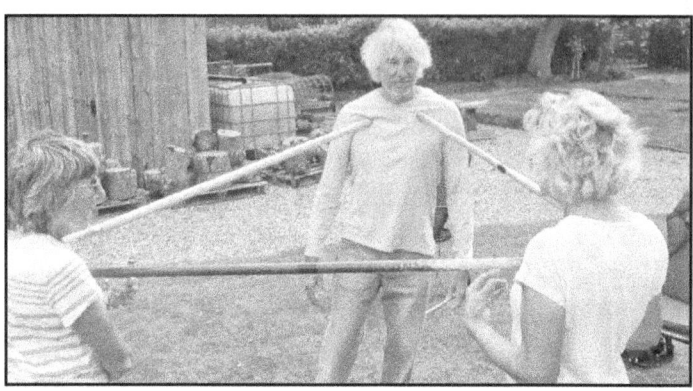

work with some contact. There are several important reasons for this:

- it helps with range

- it overcomes psychological issues of hitting and being hit

- you get used to the idea that in a fight you might get hit!

- it gives an opportunity to practice breathing and control of our psyche

- it helps develop good striking ability as opposed to always "pulling" a strike

- we learn how to gauge our hits and work at different depths of strike, we get instant feedback

Obviously, safety is a major factor - heavier contact should only be carried out once people have the mechanisms in place to deal with it. The better people are at taking hits, the heavier the hits can become. Of course there are always some areas which will be off-limits as far as power shots are concerned, unless perhaps we are using protective gear (see later on).

But even at a basic level it is important that there be at least "touch" contact. A very good method when working at this stage is to use the fist to push rather than to strike. This doesn't hurt anyone but gives valuable feedback concerning angles and positions of the strike.

Contact does not necessarily have to be related to speed. It is possible to work quite slow but with heavy strikes. Likewise, with the right kind of control, we should be able to work fast but give only surface hits. One tip to help with this is to keep the fists quite relaxed, this way we will not hit too deeply.

Contact and non-contact work can be mixed into one drill. A simple idea is for one person to try and touch the other with a stick. One is trying to get contact, the other to avoid it. I like to use gauntlet drills for this kind of work.

Another element with this variable is the idea of non-contact work. This has always been a controversial area in martial arts, particularly when it comes with claims of mysterious masters using "super-human" powers to affect others, sometimes in quite dramatic ways. That aside, the non-touch work I've experienced in Systema has always been clearly explained in psychological terms. At a basic level, we can think of this as eliciting a flinch response by putting an obstacle in the way. For example a clear flick towards the eyes or groin can affect a change in movement and structure in a person, which we can then take advantage of. This is a starting point and can lead into other areas of training, such as reading body language, affecting others through our own actions and so on.

Alongside this is "soft work". This is where we try and influence someone with a minimum of contact. This is useful in that we learn to work with minimum tension on our part, and our work does not aggravate those we are working against, making it easier to gain compliance. There are numerous close protection drills that help develop this useful skill - one that I've used several times to calm down a situation.

Touch has a powerful effect on the

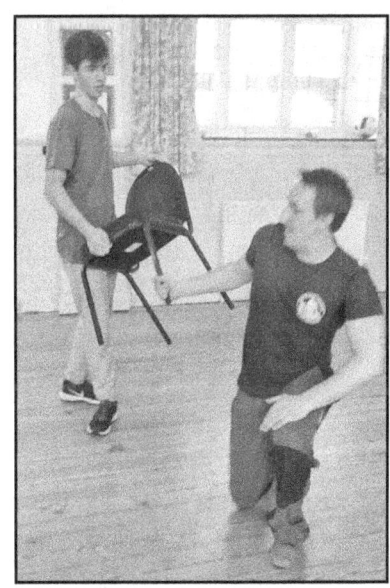

nervous system, either to calm or agitate, so a study of different contact levels is very important

POINT FOUR - TECHNIQUE

Sometimes we will practice one specific technique, either in order to explore a principle, or where some technical knowledge is required. I will talk a little more about this later on, but this is basically to allow us to concentrate solely on one particular area in order to develop skills in it.

To turn things around, we may wish to learn more about defence from a certain technique. So we set up our partner to feed in only kicks, or grabs and so on. This gives us a chance to repeatedly experience something specific and so learn a good response against it.

POINT FIVE - COMPLIANCE

Outside people are often surprised at the amount of compliance in martial arts training. They seem to think all our time is spent fighting in some sort of gladiatorial trial and that training is all about being "hard" or "tough". The reality is far different of course, in every style or method there is a considerable amount of development work prior to any kind of full contact.

This is no different to any other area of life or training. No musician plays their first gig at Wembley Arena in front of thousands of people - and if that did happen, they would be so out of their depth as to be useless. More importantly they would be unlikely to gain anything from the experience, indeed it could put them off for life!

Having said that, there is the opposite extreme, where everything you do in training works and classmates obligingly crumple at a touch. Once again, the truth lies somewhere in-between.

So how much should we resist what our partner is doing? That depends entirely on the purpose of the drill. If we take locks and holds as an example, the base level is purely to learn the actual mechanics of the technique. Then, at some point we need to know what to do if your partner resists.

There are three aspects to consider when it comes to compliance. The first is tension as resistance - our partner grabs and we can apply a lot of tension in order to counter the technique

The second is to not let the partner apply their technique in the first place, ie to be evasive. The third is to actively work back against our partner, so maybe while they are grabbing us, we punch them.

Once you have these three ideas in mind it becomes easy to start grading levels of resistance. There are two other things to consider – one is the relative level of each partner. If a person is highly skilled they may be able to stop their partner very easily. This can prove frustrating for the beginner. A good person can adjust on the

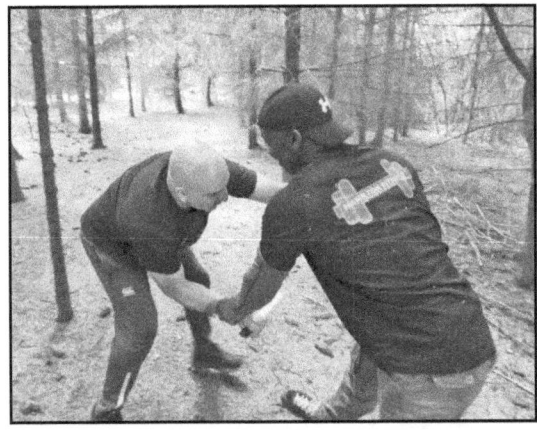

fly in order to give their partner a good training experience.

The second consideration is safety. If you have a joint put under pressure, you may be able to apply tension in order to stop it moving. However this may then give your partner a quandary – do they apply more power in order to drive their technique through if, in doing so, they may damage the joint?

Sometimes what looks like compliance is, in fact, self preservation. A person is moving, rolling or similar in order to protect themselves from their partner's technique. This partly goes back to what I said before about the better you can deal with impact, etc, the more intensely you can work.

This also goes back to my earlier point about the notion of the *uke/nage* model not being applicable to our method. It's an extremely important idea and one that I think forms the basis for a lot of the online miscomprehension of Systema videos. People assume that the person hitting is "showing off" his punches and the other partner is just a dummy. In fact, as we know, these drills are for the benefit of the person being hit, thrown, etc.

We have already mentioned the importance of avoiding getting so wrapped up in "resistance" and tension that you fail even to feel the touch of a knife or similar. It doesn't mean you have to fade at the first touch, but you must at least acknowledge the potential of what is happening to you. This process is about self awareness as much as anything else.

There is a psychological aspect to resistance, too. Training that is always done in a cool, calm, friendly environment is not necessarily preparing us for real life. People can be belligerent, aggressive, insulting, they may shout and scream at us, even if no physical harm is intended. This can have as dramatic an effect on our nervous system as any punch or kick, so it is good to cover this in training too, particularly when we get into scenario work.

Resistance levels, then, should be set according to the purposes of the drill and the relative skills of the people involved. I find that my regular guys, who have worked together for years, are able to go at high speed and resistance levels without any

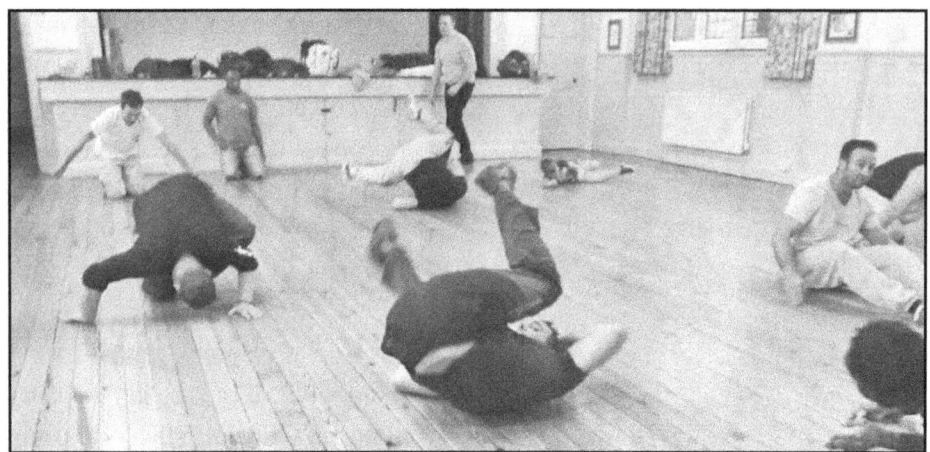

problems. We are fortunate to have had very few injuries in training over the years and I can say that those few we have had were down to people going outside of the drill boundaries.

POINT SIX - ENVIRONMENT
Environment is such an obvious variable, yet so many people train week after week in exactly the same room, they may even stand in exactly the same space and work with exactly the same people. One of the first comments about our classes is…. "there's no mats!" There are a few reasons for this. The most obvious is that 99.999% of the world is not matted – and that is where things happen.

Groundwork on a normal floor gives us much better feedback and means our bodies learn to relax so much quicker. Of course, it is uncomfortable at first, but discomfort can be a good teacher! Likewise learning to fall and dive on a normal surface teaches us good technique very quickly. This means we can adapt much easier to whatever surface we are working on.

Don't think that you should never use mats, though. There may be some circumstances with newer or very nervous people or if you are trying more daring falls, where mats can help at first. But they should be removed at the earliest opportunity so that they don't become a habit.

Whilst on the subject of ground surface, even if people don't train with mats, they tend to be on a nice wooden floor. Even working on a flat lawn can make a big difference, let alone uneven ground.

In short, vary your training space. Get outside, onto grass, concrete, woodland, anywhere and everywhere. Now, this does open a question as to the viability of training outside in the UK. I find that even training "normal" exercise outside attracts attention here - whereas in the Far East public spaces are full of people training everything from Taijii to ballroom dancing. So you have to pick your spots carefully. It bears consideration, especially if you are thinking of using training weapons. If you are not in a public space, make sure you get permission from the land owner, unless you want to run an evasion drill as we once did in a park after closing time.....

There are many types of environment to work in – a car or vehicle of some kind, narrow corridor, different rooms, stairs and so on. Take a look around your training space. If you are in a local hall, you may find stairs, a kitchen, toilets, a car park, a stage, all good potential training areas.

Environment can also cover sound - try training with different types and volumes of music. It can refer to the number of people around. If you have a large group, put them in a small room and get them to move through and around, or work group sparring. With a very large group you can work some good crowd drills. Don't just think "fighting", any of these drills may help if you are somewhere and there is an emergency situation. Remember Systema training is for survival, not just for a fight!

POINT SEVEN - RESTRICTION
Adding restriction to a drill is done for two reasons. It can be to simulate a situation where you are not fully functional due to injury, are carrying something or are restricted due to environment. It can also be in order to focus on a specific sense or area of the body.

Restriction is most simply done by taking one or more parts of the body out of the equation. So you might work with hands in pockets, standing on one leg, carrying some object, having to work on the spot and so on. Blindfold work is extremely useful in this respect. It develops tactile sensitivity, general awareness, intuitive feeling and is good for fear control. Group blindfold exercises also teach teamwork, trust and communication skills

There are other aspects to working with restriction. There may be a situation where it is not appropriate for you to hit someone, so you have to work within the restriction of trying to restrain them only. Restriction can also apply to time - giving a drill a specific length can be useful in some cases, especially testing or task related drills.

POINT EIGHT - EQUIPMENT
Equipment can refer to regular sparring gear – gloves, head guards, padding, gum shields and so on. We have found there are pros and cons to using them. On the plus side, it allows for higher levels of speed and contact. On the down side we find it can restrict breathing and vision, allows a person to continue despite heavy hits and gives a different sense of distance if large gloves are worn.

Of course, you don't have to be totally

covered. We sometime use light bag gloves as hand protection for faster sparring, which generally works well. Something else we use are focus pads. Again,they have pros and cons but can be very useful for helping people develop flow and power in their strikes.

For some areas of training though, protective gear is compulsory - for example, eye protection if using airsoft or fast weapon work. However we have found that this type of equipment has little or no effect on the actual work.

Equipment doesn't just mean protective gear though. Perhaps the single most useful bit of equipment for Systema training is a stick – there are are huge amount of stick exercises for solo, partner and group work.

When it comes to exercise some people like to use sledgehammers, kettlebells, an iron ball, logs, power bands and similar for training. Again, this gives us the opportunity to be creative and not just think "gym weights" for training strength.

Weapons are part of almost all martial arts training. There are numerous benefits to learning the use of and defence against all types of weapon, be it bladed, blunt or projectile. We can think of "proper" weapons, such as knife and also "improvised" weapons, everyday items that may be used in some way, such as a chair, items of clothing etc.

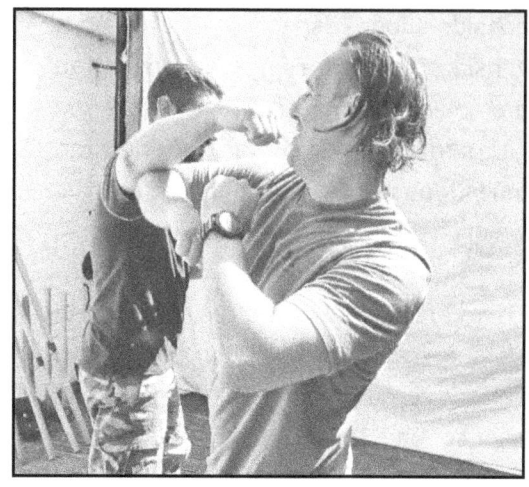

POINT NINE - PURPOSE

It is absolutely vital in training that we are aware of why we do what we do. It is very easy to slip into a comfortable routine, even in Systema . We have already spoken about lesson plans, but regardless of wether you use them or not, it is important to understand the main purpose of drills that you are setting up.

Another aspect to this is the question of balance. I've been in pre-Systema classes where one particular aspect of the training becomes (to my mind) over-emphasised. A prime example is the push-hands training we see in some styles. What begins as a useful exercise for developing tactile awareness, structure and technique becomes almost the whole point of the training. The criteria for effectiveness then becomes how good you are at a particular drill rather than how well you can use the skills developed from it in real life. We should always understand the purpose of restrictions in training is not to just be able to work under those restrictions!

Training for a specific event or sport means we are able to focus our efforts towards that goal. The same goes for a person training for a particular role, such as a doorman. It is when we start training for "self defence" that things can become less clear. In any kind of drill, then, it is important to have a clearly defined reason for the drill. I have divided these into seven categories:

Play
An enjoyable exchange between two or more people. The main goal is simply to enjoy the movement and be "in the moment". It gives a chance to be creative and try out new ideas or movements in a relaxed environment.

Attribute Development
Some attributes to consider are balance, visual awareness, tactile sensitivity, emotional awareness, flow, reactions, speed, team work, confidence, communication, fear management, co-ordination, fine and gross motor skills, health and so on.

Learning
The aim here is to learn or refine a new technical skill, or how to work with some piece of equipment. Work is restricted solely to the technique or skill in question

Testing
Once we have some skills we need to test them. Trying to hit a moving opponent, testing movement skills against a weapon and so on. In each case there should be a clearly defined "succeed or fail" element built in so you can gauge how your skills held up!

Problem Solving
Problem solving might be as simple as being put into an arm-bar, then working out how to escape from it. It might be how to move and protect a person through a group of attackers. Generally this type of drill will be run at less than full speed with plenty of time to work things out

Task Based
Similar to Problem Solving but in "real time". The task might be to pin a person to the floor for five seconds. Or it could be to prevent someone getting through a doorway, extracting

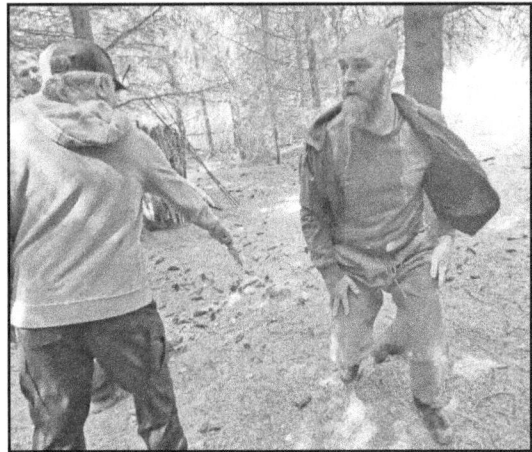

someone from a car and so on. There will usually be a time limit in place to keep things focused.

Simulation

In essence this means creating some kind of scenario or role-play in order to simulate a real life situation. They can be very simple, or quite involved.

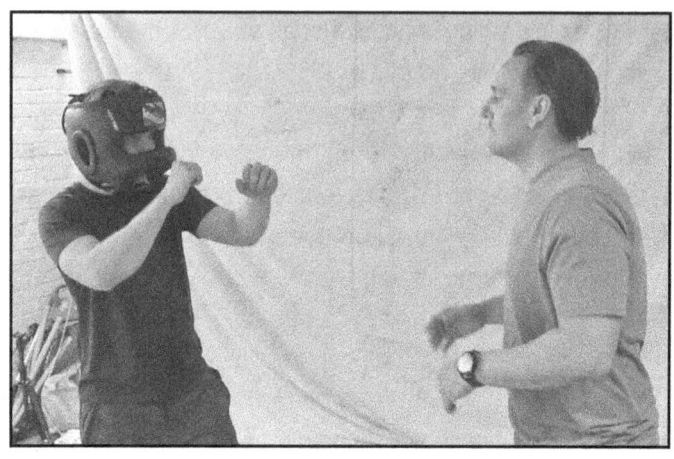

Scenario work also brings in the idea of pre, during and post incident considerations. There may be a build up to physical action, which gives a good opportunity to develop fear control. As we know, any physical action needs to be appropriate to the situation, or post-incident consequences may be dire. I see some schools practicing neck breaks and kicks to the head of a downed attacker. Appropriate in some cases perhaps, but in others, you will be in the dock alongside your attacker. As an instructor, you should always do your best to pass on sound knowledge of local law and other potential consequences.

POINT TEN - INTENSITY

Our final variable is how we blend all the other variables together! They can and should be mixed and matched in almost countless ways in order to enhance the training experience. As I mentioned, think of the variables as a graphic equaliser - each band can be adjusted individually until the mix is just how you like it.

This brings a huge amount of variety into our training and helps prevent lessons becoming stale and too comfortable. The whole training session can even be built around virtually the same drill run in a variety of ways. For example, start with knife handling, then go to close-in flow knife-disarming, build up speed to test, work in some problem solving with the knife held close in a restricted space, then finish with some scenario work based on some real life knife attack situations.

The important thing is that everyone is aware of the drill boundaries and the purposes of the drill - and I often find we discover some other purposes as we go along! Also, the drill is always open to change and adaptation as and when necessary.

TECHNIQUE OR PRINCIPLE?

Systema is known for primarily taking a principle-based approach. I've even heard people say "there are no techniques in System!". Well, yes, in an ideal world. But we have to be realistic and we have to start from where people are, not where we would like them to be. I had an example of exactly this just recently, with some students who, while by no means new to class, struggled throughout a set of drills with what I was showing them. My frustration must have become evident as one of them even mentioned it!

Was this their fault or mine? To me, the work was quite basic and obvious, yet both struggled to apply it. It made me go away and think about the particular work and how I presented it. So next session we did the same work, only this time I broke the movements down into four basic techniques - inside-up, inside-down, outside-up, outside-down. This worked much better for them, they were able to get into the swing of the drill. The session after, we were able to freestyle much more, as had been my original intention.

So never be afraid to drop back to technique if it is required. In fact, for some of the more technical aspects of work, such as locks, I'd always advise starting with some basic techniques. Sometimes, people want to go away from class feeling they have actually learned something. It is an interesting bit of psychology.

When I first began adding bits of Systema into my previous teaching, I actually tried an experiment. I had two groups at the time. One I told "tonight we are going to learn the move White Crane Cools its Wings." There was an actual "ooooh!" went round the group. In the other session, I said "lets do some work against close in punches and grabs."

I showed both groups exactly the same movements. One in a broken down, step by step way, the other more freeform. I found that the first group quickly felt confident with the move, they had a certainty about having learned this particular technique. When everything was set in place, it worked great - yet they struggled much more applying it in a live drill.

The second group had no real thought of "knowing" something, yet were able to apply the method consistently well in free sparring. It was an interesting lesson for me and one that nudged me further along the Systema path.

Unfortunately, when it comes to marketing, or promoting that "feel good" factor about your sessions, selling certainty largely wins out, particularly in the mainstream. I seen endless self defence clips of "what to do if…" They present some magic move or technique, with no thought as to the actual attributes required to make it work. It is the same in my health work. I've had people ask me "how can I deal with my stress?" I answer along the lines of "take ten minutes a day to do these breathing exercises as a start." The response is sometimes "I'm way too busy to do that." So they may often end up never dealing with the stress, or get into some type of pill or medication, with its associated problems.

All that aside, if you find students are struggling with principles, drop back to technique. Remember all those other tools we have too, time slicing, working slowly and so on. The aim is to present our information in digestible chunks, and that will vary from person to person. The challenge in a group is often pitching the learning at the median level. Go too low and more experienced get bored. Go too high and newer people struggle. This is where the concept of everyone doing the same drill at different levels kick in. And there is nothing wrong with giving a more experienced pair some leeway in the drill you have set, or tell them they can work faster, or apply more subtle work.

CREATING A DRILL

Thanks to training with the top teachers, plus access to downloads and Youtube clips, instructors have a ton of drills that we can use "out of the box." However, this shouldn't prevent us from either tweaking those drills, as mentioned, or making up our own. You may sometimes be in a position where you have to make a drill up on the spot. This usually happens to me when I ask "what do you want to practice today?" And someone responds with "well, this happened to me last week, how should I have managed it?"

I like this type of drill best as it relates directly to a person's experience, plus we can incorporate what they actually did in the situation - if it was successful!

One of the cornerstones of Systema is creativity and adaptability in training, and we have discussed many ways to tweak an existing drill, but what are the principles and guidelines for creating your own? The first thing to consider is the purpose of the drill. This may be very specific - for example I want people to learn how to work against a knife held to the

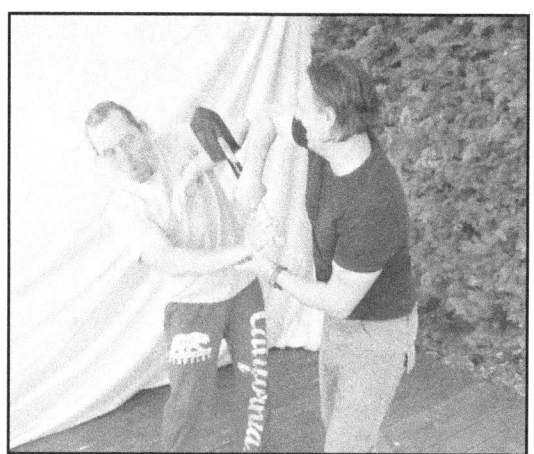

throat. Or it may be more general, such as I want to get people moving about. As we have said, often there will be more than one benefit from doing the drill, but focus first on that primary aim. Once you have the purpose of the drill look at the factors that will shape it.

Basic set up - who does what and under what conditions?

Effective - is the drill effective in delivering the result?

Practical - is it practical to run the drill in your training environment; do you have the necessary space, conditions, equipment, knowledge? Do you have sufficient people to run the drill?

Safety - what are the risks of injury and how can they be minimised whilst keeping the drill realistic?

Understandable - how easy is it for students to understand the purpose and boundaries of the drill? While it is good for students to discover some things for yourself it is also good that they at least some notion of why they are doing a particular drill. The only exception may be those drills that have a surprise element..

Supervision - will you be able to adequately supervise the drill, watch for people going outside of the boundaries, and tweak on the fly? Is there a mechanism in place where you can stop the drill immediately if needed?

Adaptability - can the drill be tweaked as it goes along?

Two way learning - is the drill beneficial for everyone involved, not just "attacker vs defender?

Challenge - what is the level of challenge for students involved? Too much can be as bad as not enough. Can pressure be increased / decreased as necessary during the drill?

Progression - can the drill be expanded upon, or extra layers added in?

So let's put all this into practice and invent a drill. Once you have read this, grab a pen and paper and invent your own!

Purpose - to increase students awareness of how knives are carried / hidden.

Basic structure - group of 12 students. Three are carrying a hidden knife, nine are spotters. The students move normally around the training area, each has to spot who is carrying a knife.

Effective - this mirrors how knives are often carried in deployed in street situations, so should provide some useful skills of awareness and avoidance.

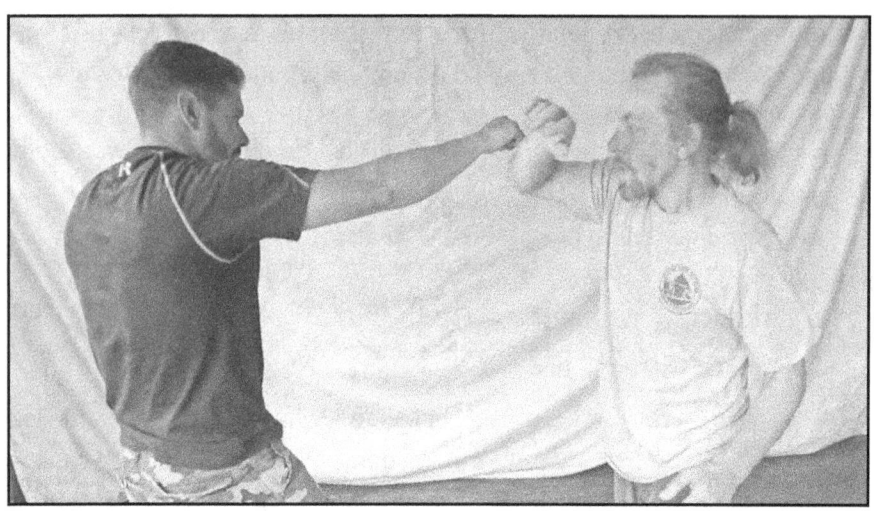

Practical - needs a certain amount of space, can be indoor or outdoor, furniture or obstacles can be added. Equipment required - training knives, maybe eye protection.

Safety - use of training knives only, no metal blades. Care taken not to stab to the face unless there is eye protection.

Understandable - role and restrictions should be clearly explained, it is all quite straightforward,

Supervision - quite easy to move around the edge of the group and keep an eye on things. Use a whistle to stop and start the drill.

Adaptability - will include speed of movement, amount of space, low light levels, increase / decrease the number of knives available.

Two way learning - one group are learning to watch for and avoid the hidden knife. The other are learning about concealment and deployment of the knife.

Challenge - can be easily ramped up or down as required. It is good to up the intensity at some point to give some experience of a real life situation. At those levels, everyone will get "cut", which is a secondary purpose of the drill - to highlight the danger and difficulty of this type of work.

Progressions - knife holders draw knife and make a single attack at random which must be avoided or checked.

As above but continuous attack from knife holder until subdued or target is stabbed three or four times.

As above but the spotters can work as a team when a knife come out to subdue the attacker.

Hopefully you will see that once you have the broad outline and function of the drill, it is easy to go back over all those modifiers we mentioned before and add them in. This gives you great freedom as an instructor to explore any aspect of training that you wish.

Given the resources, you can do anything. Want to work in water? Hire as local swimming pool as we have done and run drills there. Or you may have access to a bus, or a bar, or explore methods of safely restraining people. You may even just want to have a bit of fun with sword fighting, or stunt work or free running, all are possible with a little planning.

The only the caveat with "application" drills are that things must remain practical and realistic. That doesn't mean every drill has to involve a pseudo life-and-death struggle full of drama and tension, but that each drill must effectively deliver results beyond itself. We all have favourite drills, but don't hang on to them like a comfort blanket.

Always remember drills are not the goal of the training, they just something to use on the way to wherever you are going!

CHAPTER EIGHT
CLASS CONTENT

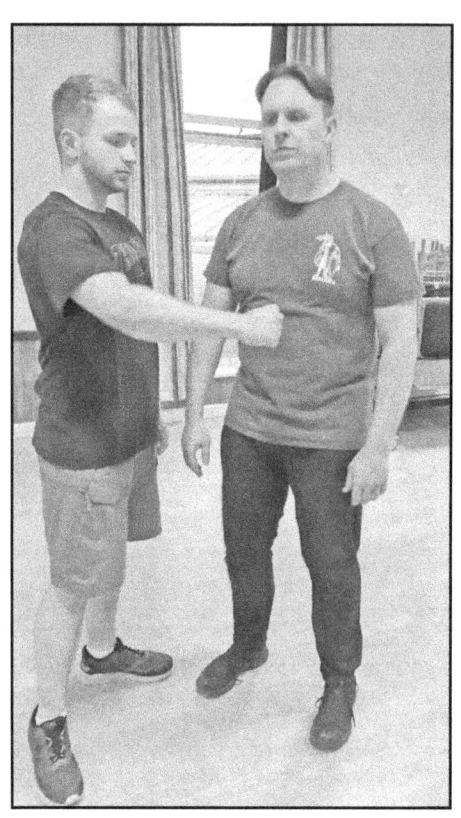

Let's next look at ideas for actual content for your classes. Now, it would take several volumes to detail every single possible drill, and I have, of course, described a wide range of drills in previous books. What I will do here, then, is give you some ideas for fundamental drills for new students. From there, we will look at some more subtle work and deeper levels, plus ideas on setting up sparring, testing and scenario drills. We have covered the numerous ways we can tweak these drills in the previous chapter, so I shall restrict myself here to explaining only the base level, or broad outline of each.

FUNDAMENTALS

While there is no set syllabus in Systema, there are certain key requirements students need in order to be able to train properly. So if you are starting a class for the very first time, with a group of new people, the following should give you a good few months of work and your students a strong foundation.

Don't ever be worried about returning to the "basics." My view is that there isn't really such a thing as basic and advanced work, they are all different expressions of the same thing. Systema is not so much about progression through performing more and more intricate movements. In fact, it is more about simplifying what we do through refinement and deeper understanding. As the saying goes, "with the best master, you see very little." In that sense, we all need to go back to "basic" drills now and then just to check ourselves.

Breathing

Virtually every class I run, on whatever topic and with whatever group, starts with breathing. For the most part I use the selective tension exercise from earlier. This puts everyone in touch with their breathing, allows them to feel relaxation and brings them into the mental space required for the class ahead.

The next thing is to teach the four depths of breathing;
Burst / recovery - in/out, shallow
Upper chest - expands a little on in breath
Full chest - deeper into the lungs, shoulders pull back a little, chest expands
Diaphragm - belly breathing either normal or reverse (don't rush into this too quickly)

Next comes breath control. I used a combination of shapes and numbers for this.

Circle - inhale/exhale equal
Triangle - inhale/hold/exhale equal
Square - inhale /hold/exhale/hold equal
Rectangle - inhale / longer hold / exhale / longer hold

Simple count - eg 4 in, 4 out
Ladders - progression, so 2 in, 2 out
4 in 4 out
6 in 6 out

8 in 8 out
10 in 10 out
Then back down the ladder

Finally, for now, breath holds and recovery. These can be static at first, later add in some movement or exercise.
Inhale and hold for long as possible.
Exhale and hold for as long as possible
Explain how to pinpoint and release any internal tension whilst holding.
Recovery breath, stress the importance of fully recovering both breath and heart rate

Also look at integration. So you might combine ladders with square breathing patterns. Look then at wider integration, tying the breath work into the physical activity, be it exercise or drill.

Falling

You'd be surprised at the number of people practicing martial arts that don't learn to fall well. Obviously in some styles, such as Judo, it is a major part of the training, though often the "slap the ground" type of work which is not always applicable outside of the dojo.

With some exceptions, it's rare to see even a basic level of training in falls, let alone work at the level of the Systema approach. To me, managing falls is a skill that goes way beyond martial arts in any case - it is a true "self defence" and life skill that we will all need at some point!

In my opinion Systema teaches the safest and practical ways to fall. We don't rely on breakfalls, for example, or teach people to accelerate into a throw. Likewise, our concern is always that practice should be good for the body, not damaging it, so the stress is always on relaxation and blending.

It may be one of the most important but I'd bet money on falling being the most unpopular aspect of training! I certainly struggled with it, coming from a background where the response to "how do I fall?" was "you don't fall, you stay on your feet."

The first challenge is overcoming the fear of falling and the best way to do that, is start on the ground. This gradated approach, gradually increasing the height of the fall, works very well to overcome fears and tensions. I've worked this successfully not only with my self defence groups, but also with elderly people too. Here's the basic outline. The work is on mats, if available.

Lay down on your back and get comfortable.
Run through some breath work.
Feel what mobility you have in this position. Move your arms and legs, twist around a little. See if you can use your shoulders to shuffle around a bit.
Roll onto your side - do this by threading one foot under and through the opposite knee and turning the hips.
Roll onto your back. Do this by leading with your top hand/arm

From your back, inhale, then exhale and sit up. Inhale and go back down again.

This sequence should help relax the body and get people comfortable with being on the ground. Time for Stage Two.

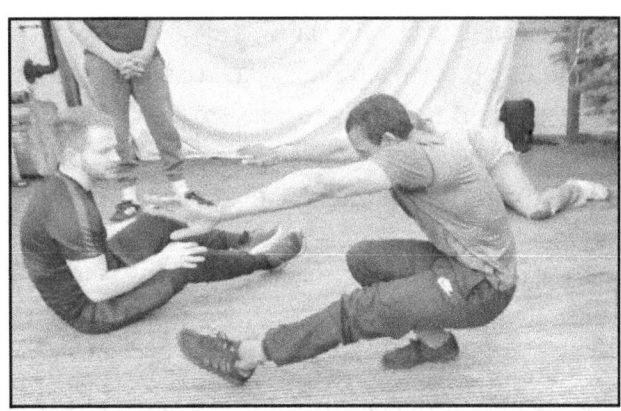

Sit up again. Place a hand out to the side, palm down, and ease your weight into it a little.

Explain how when people fall, they often put out a hand to stop the fall, usually resulting in injury to the wrist or arm. This is what we call *bracing*.

Instead we employ the principle of *sliding*. Sit and place the hand out to the side again. This time, as the weight goes into that arm, the hand slides out and back a little. This should slowly bring the body down onto its side.

Stress the exhale/relax connection.

Repeat on each side. Slide onto the side, sit up.

Now perform as a continuous movement. Slide, body down, wiggle the shoulders to shift the weight across to the opposite side, sit up.

This should give you a kind of circular sit up type movement that will not only gently strengthen the core but will reinforced the concept of sliding when the hand touches the floor. Contrast it with break-falling, which may be problematic when not working on mats.

Something you can also add in is to have the free hand cup the back of the head on the fall, in order to protect it. Always stress the need to fall onto the soft parts of the body rather than the bony areas!

The progression from here is simply to increase the height. So, work from a kneeling position, a squat, and finally standing.

That is falling back, but how about forward? I start this work against a wall. The person stands a couple of feet away and falls forward. Bring out the palms and, as they contact the wall, bend the elbows, a bit like doing a press up. This is to introduce us to the concept of *folding*. Again, we may be starting in a brace position, but we relax the arm off to absorb the impact.

Next, contact and bend just one arm. Let's say it's the right. Fall forward, right arm extends, palm touches the wall. Bend the right elbow and turn the body a little. This will bring the right shoulder to the wall. Continue the movement, rolling against the wall onto your back. Step away.

So the impact of the fall is now neutralised by the arm folding and the rolling movement. We are not hitting the wall head on. Stress how the folding movement helps slow the body down, so lessening impact.

Once people have the idea, go back to the floor and have them try it from a push up position. Lower, fold the arm, roll to the side and push back up again. From there, we have the same progression of working from knees, squat and standing.

The final solo drill at this level, is to have a person stand and gradually change their stance. So they widen the feet out, lean the body a little and so on. The aim is to bring the body as close to the floor before falling. This is a very nice one as the faller retains control of when and how they fall. Following this, you can shift into partner work, confident that everyone can manage at least a basic fall or throw.

Movement

We need to consider mobility while both upright and on the ground. For the first, stick drills always work very well. They give a clear line of movement, and allow a little time to respond. They are also teaching the wielder how to use a stick, and some of its basic movement patterns.

A and B stand about a stick's length distance apart. A will move the stick in set patterns. B has to avoid contact with it Think of the four types of movement.

Thrust - A pushes one end of the stick out. B twists or steps to the side to avoid.

Dropping - the stick is held upright at one end and A lets it drop forward. B steps to one side to avoid.

Swinging - A swings the stick in an arc. This can be done at three heights. Head height, B ducks under. Mid-height, B steps back to avoid. Ankle height - B jumps over the stick.

Diagonal - A swings the stick in a diagonal upward or downward strike. B moves in, out or ducks under to avoid. If A makes this strike continuous, they will be working into the Figure 8 pattern.

Start with each movement clear and slow. Progress to faster (but still safe), then begin to mix the movements up, make them more random. A can also explore different angles or ways to wield the stick.

This drill gives a good basic understanding of integrated movement - if one part is left behind, it gets hit! That will help with posture and, of course, we always stress the exhale/relax/move connection. There is also a very clear success / failure indicator, as the only goal is to avoid contact with the stick! Again, this simple drill forms the basis for much of the later work.

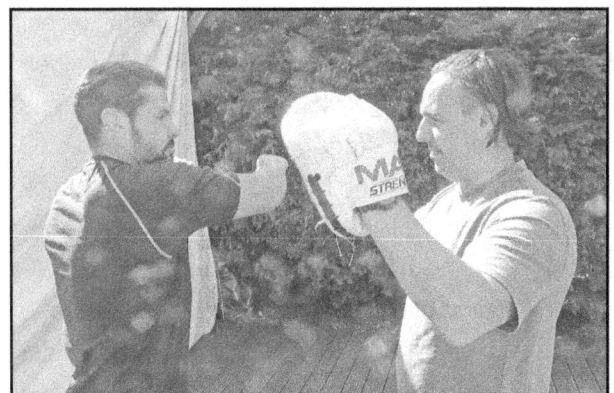

If students have done the falling work, they already some idea of ground movement. Simply take the first part of that training and expand on it. Have people moving in the ground using only their shoulders, legs, arms, etc, on their front side and back.

For partner work, A moves on the ground and B simply walks towards them. This can be a large movement at first, you can use counting steps to set this. So B takes ten steps in a straight line, then turns, lines up on B and takes ten steps again. B's only job is to avoid contact. Then decrease the number of steps B takes, so giving A less time to think.

Strikes

I usually start new people off on the pads with a basic Figure 8 pattern to start. Use a single pad at first, have them slap into it with a downward diagonal strike - so right hand up high, drop it down and across to the left into the pad. Be sure the pad is held at the right angle. This gets the student into using their waist to twist into the hit and also the idea of dropping weight into the lead leg too. Emphasise breathing and the fact that they should not be putting any power in at this stage, keep the arm relaxed, this is about movement.

Repeat on both sides. Now work two pads. The slap down into one, then bring the hand back up to hammer fist the opposite pad. Slow at first, but you can work this into a sharp 1-2 movement. Repeat on both sides.

The next stage is to make that move more continuous. In other words, the hands are working in a figure 8, one closely following the other. We are now getting two hits into each pad, one directly after the other. The sound should be a little like a train! Ba-da, ba-da, ba-da. Start slow and gradually speed up. If the student loses place, re-set and start slow again.

As always, mention the breathing. This is a good one to work with breath counts, or even ladder breaths and holds/ recovery. Once a person can hit the pads in a smooth, crisp and powerful Figure 8 pattern, they have a good foundation to get into some of the other types of striking.

Incidentally, after working pads I always like to run a drill or two on the application of the movement we have just been doing. It stops the pad work becoming too abstract - unless you are running more of a fitness class, in which case they are great for developing coordination and cardio too!

The other side of strikes work is learning to take them. We covered the foundation method for this before, plus I again refer you to Vladimir's excellent *Strikes* book

Takedowns
An important tool and a great chance to practice both structure breaking and managing falls! We already mentioned the 3D concept before, which is an ideal intro drill .

Knifework
I like to start knifework by first having students handle a knife. This can be a training blade, metal is best. Simply have them move the knife around, change grips and so on. Show them how to work with the flat of the blade to change the knife position, switch grips and so on. This builds familiarity with the knife, both on a physical and psychological level.

From there, we start by having A lightly press the point of the training knife into B's body. B goes with the direction of the movement, and moves away. This can by with the whole body, by stepping, or by just rotating the area touched. This is quite a regular drills for us as it gets people to relax very quickly.

Next, B moves just enough to deflect the point, pins A's wrist with one hand, then strips the knife out with the other. Stress that at this stage we are working with only one part of the body, the hand. Refer back to our time slice concept.

The next stage is to extend the work out to the rest of A. So now, once the knife is neutralised, B can work into locks, holds, takedowns and so on. From there you can begin to add in more movement, or work in multiples.

An important thing to always point out when doing knife work in particular is that all our work is based on the principle of damage limitation. That damage is initially to me, of course! Martial arts are full of amazing techniques to take the knife or gun, to choke out attackers and so on. Systema is

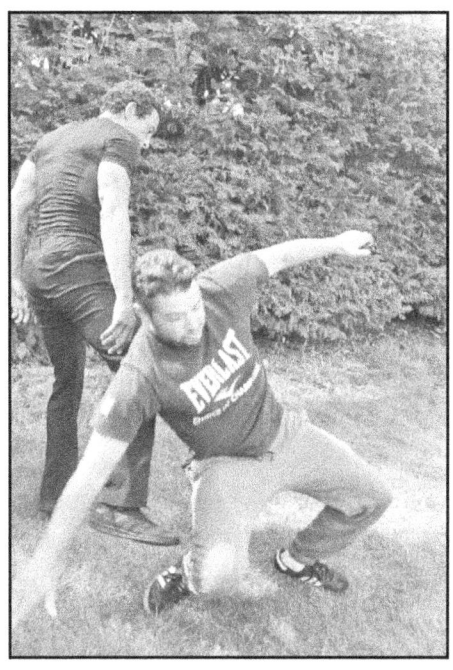

one of the few that asks "but what if that doesn't work?" This is the main reason we work from principle - if something is not working and we understand the principles, we can alter things on the fly.

If all we have is rote technique, then typically, if it doesn't work first time, people keep trying to reapply the same thing over and over. In Systema, we adapt and flow, there is no hang up on performance, it is all about result.

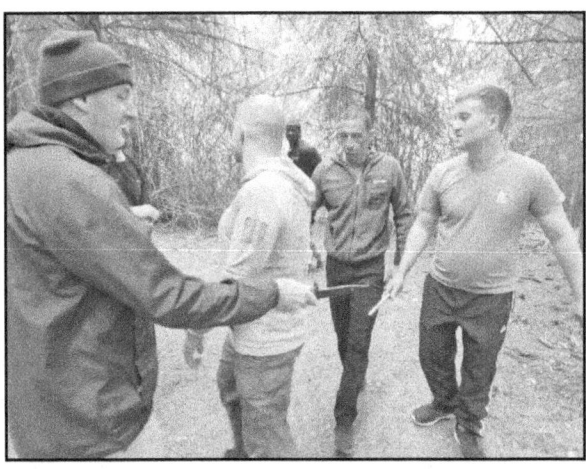

I bring this up in particular with knife work as people can look at our drills and think "that technique will never work" when, in fact, what they are seeing is usually attribute development rather than a knife attack simulation. And one of those attributes is learning what to do when things go wrong. I mean, in a way, if the knife is that close, things have already gone wrong. So how do you deal with it?

I'm reminded of time when I taught at a multi-style event and opened with this drill, starting with knife contact. One person loudly proclaimed "but I'd never let the knife get that close!" I mentioned some incidents I'd been involved in and also pointed to the numerous CCTV examples of real knife attacks.

That person remained sceptical until, later on, we did the knives in a crowd drill, where everyone gets stabbed at some point. Then the penny dropped. But it was interesting and alarming to me to hear such an attitude from a martial artist. Having such a belief in your abilities and techniques is quite dangerous, potentially fatally so.

So always stress the damage limitation aspect and also the fact that sometimes we use the knife merely as point of focus. For example, we were running a drill with the military shovel recently, how to use the handle end. We worked against a knife purely because it gave a nice, clear attack to work with, to help the students get familiarity with using the shovel. The aim of the drill was not knife defence - though, of course, it builds attributes that are useful in knife defence, which we can try out in our testing phase..

Groundwork

The last foundation area we will look it is fighting on the ground. We have already covered some ground movement, now the idea is to put some of those movements into actual application. Here, we should also include ways of quickly and safely getting back up again.

There are broadly two situations in ground fighting - you on the ground and them standing, or everyone on the ground. Let's start with the first, and some work against kicks and stamps.

A lays down. B applies pressure to various parts of B's body with the foot. A's job is to escape out from the pin with minimal movement.

From there, A moves into following up the escape with a takedown, usually working against B's knees or ankles. Next, add in some movement, have B stepping in to apply the stamp. B can now work a little earlier, or wait for the contact.

The same procedure works for kicks. B starts by placing the foot (B can be sitting now) and pushing. B first learns to accept and move with the push. Next, they build a response into the escape movement, working against either the supporting or the pushing leg. Finally, add in the movement as before.

For actual ground grappling, start with A simply putting their weight across B, who must wriggle out from underneath. From there, show a couple of simple pins for A to apply, and how B can best escape from them. This work then easily progresses to various types of locks and hold. You will probably find this work starts off with technique, but always be sure to explain the underlying principles. Also, think back to our three time ranges. Explore escaping from locks before, during and after they are applied.

Grappling is the easiest type of work to set up sparring, as people can work with decent levels of intensity without too much risk. Obviously, students need to be aware of their partners safety. People sometimes question why in Systema we rarely, if ever, "tap out". This is where you tap a hand on the floor or yourself to indicate that "you got me, let's start again," or "if you apply that lock any harder you'll break my arm!"

While it can be useful in some circumstances, tapping is not something we encourage for a couple of reasons.

First, it should be obvious to your partner that the joint is under extreme pressure and doesn't need any more. This should be apparent by feel, but also listen to your partner's breathing. If they go into burst breathing, which they should do if under stress, that is a sign you might need to halt or ease off.

Second, we can get into a habit of tapping too quickly, and also of letting go if someone taps - which I have seen done

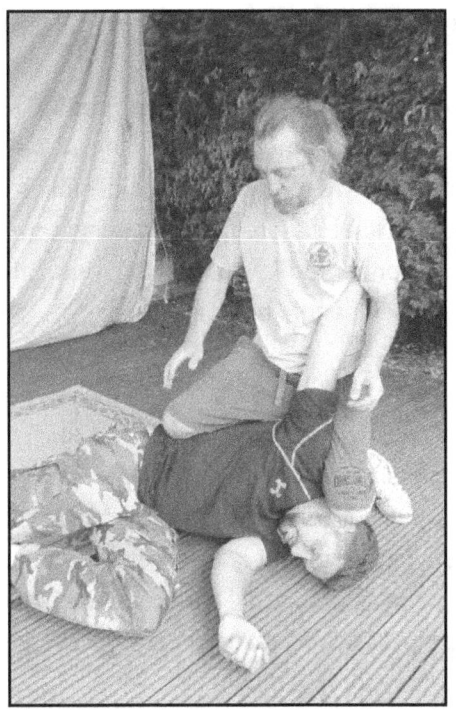

in a street fight, much to the regret of the grappler. So, when a lock or hold really does bite, burst breath to deal with any tension, then ask your partner not to release it, but to hold it there. This is where, as an instructor, you can offer some tips on ways to get out of this difficult situation.

There are escapes and counters to every hold, but there are also ways of thinking outside the box that can be surprisingly effective, too. Remember, we are not bound by anything here other than the framework of the drill, so explore all opportunities.

Perhaps the funniest example of these I've seen recently, was a counter to a rear naked choke. The defender simply got out their Bic lighter and applied the flame to the attacker's arm. Job done!

INTEGRATION

There are many other areas of training but the above is a good base to start from should give you a good six months of work across regular weekly classes. If you have a completely new group you may try, as I did once, to run the work in modules - so one month on strikes, one on groundwork and so on - or you can mix it all in across the sessions.

At some stage, however, we need to being work on integrating all these different aspects together. This is something I am always aware of and always looking for different ways to apply. I'm very conscious than when we do most of our drills, we are highlighting maybe only two or three aspects of a situation. We are constrained by the purpose of the drill, which is natural when we are learning specific skills or attributes - that's how everyone works.

But we also need to put those skills into the wider context to make sure they integrate with our general approach. This is one criticism I have of the multi-style approach, of boxing for hands, BJJ for grappling, etc. How do these things integrate?

Some styles are virtual polar opposites in approach, so it's rarely a case of just stringing the "best" techniques together - because techniques are nothing without the underlying principles.

My answer for regular classes is to build in integrative drills at the end of each session. Explaining this will give me the opportunity to show the structure of a full typical class. Generally, I'm looking to maintain a continuity of themes throughout, while working in different layers of training. The first thing, then, is to decide on the theme of the session. Let's take a recent example, from last week in fact, and look at working with the knees. Here's how that class went, from start to finish.

Students arrive, usual chat, especially as not seen one guy for a few weeks. As we chat we get into some stick work - basic stretching, twisting, rotation, etc

Breath work - the chat stops as we move into standing square breathing with selective tension

Hammer work - I like to include some strength training, so next up was exercises with the sledgehammers, around six movements each repeated about a dozen times.

Core exercises - 15 squats, sit ups, press ups, fairly slow, with breathing

Explain we are working with the knees, so we first do some hip rotations and figure eight movements with the knee.

Apply those moves to focus pads. Our partner holds them at just below waist height. Aim is to get at least two strikes in with the knee before putting the foot down. Not concerned with power, just the placement, angle and movement.

To work power, we hold a thicker pad against the leg and knee into it. The emphasis is on working at close range, with minimal movement. In other words, this isn't the typical "straight knee blast" that needs to go back and forth. Instead we work from the hip, twisting the knee in and up, or lifting the knee to drop down.

Once everyone can generate decent power, we work on position. A steps in with a grab or punch, B evades it and applies the knee strike (as a touch). We explore methods of stepping, how to position the body and so on.

From there, we explore the static use of the knee in takedowns. The lead foot is hooked round the attacker's lead foot, then the knee applies pressure into the attacker's shin / knee in order to make them fall. Slow work, with the emphasis on placement and position again.

Also explore the option to footsweep from this position, getting the timing right of applying the sweep just a little before the foot touches down.

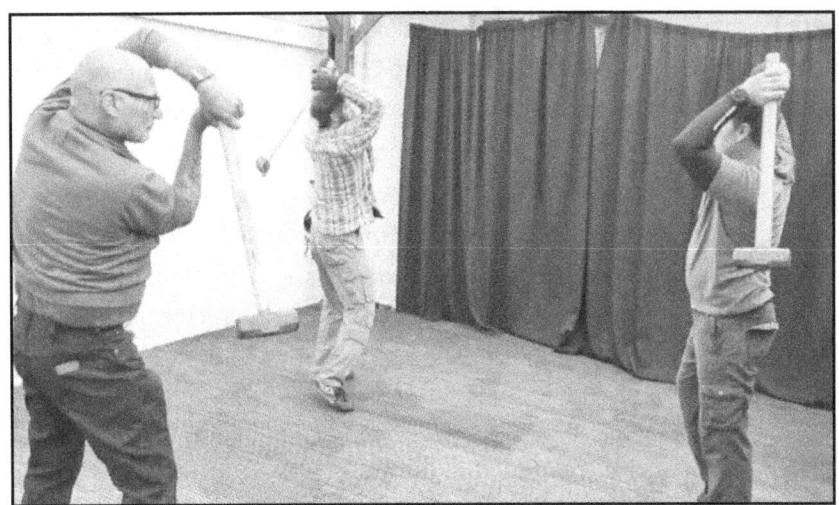

Next, working both of the above against a grab or punch, with a little more speed and aliveness. Take care as, with a little extra speed and power, you can damage your partner.

A couple more exercises - squats in particular, with emphasis on form.

Final section, free play or sparring work. We now look to work the above skills into a more free-flowing environment, so both partners can use punches, kicks, grabs, etc Newer students work under advisement, more experience students have own choice as to speed, levels of contact, use of protective gear and so on. As an instructor I keep an eye on what's going on, offer advice where needed but generally let things play out as they will.

We finish up with a 20 count push up and a circle up chat and feedback. One thing that came out during sparring was an issue of not being able to hook the foot for the takedowns. I explained how you should not chase your partner's foot, but either work where it lands or, even better, pull your partner in some way to make them step - then you know exactly where the foot is going to be.

That session ran for around 90 minutes, without any break. It was a hot day, but students grab a glug of water were they need to. I prefer to keep things moving quite briskly, though am always prepared to slow down in case of any difficulties or if something needs deeper explanation. The class level was mixed, though mostly experienced, and the work was all straightforward, though we are always looking to refine our work, to make it more subtle.

REFINEMENT

Before we move on, I want to pick up on

something I mentioned above, the question of refinement or making our work more subtle. This is where our work should go once people have the basics down. When it comes to self defence or combatives training, I tend to see a lot of emphasis on solid base techniques, but little beyond that.

This is shame because, at the risk of repeating myself, it is the attributes that develop and increase levels of skill and understanding. From the perspective of an instructor, it is vital to understand this, for three main reasons.

One, without refinement, there is no increase in skill.

Two, increase in skill leads to increase in efficiency, less chance of injury to self or others, and the ability to train with more intensity.

Three, it is this refinement that provides the Systema student with a lifetime of training, learning and growth. This is what keeps people coming to class, not doing the same old same old year in, year out.

How we go about that refinement is a big question. What I would say, though, is that you can't teach it unless you know it. So if your own work is full of tension, staccato movements and anger, that is what your students will learn. People pick up on skill in the same way they pick up on nervousness or bullshit. If your work is refined, to some degree, that will come across in your manner and in your teaching.

In other words, you need to keep up your own training. I've seen a few people who become an instructor in an art and then disappear, never to return to training. You often hear that they are teaching for a while, then the group folds. It will do. We can only teach up to our own skill level, largely. Once that point is reached, people may stay with you or, if they feel they are not developing, they may drop out.

So it is important, then, to make sure you are getting at least some level of instruction yourself. Not only will this help you develop, it will also bring you lots of new ideas to add into your own classes. Every single time I've trained with Vladimir, be it live or on Zoom, I've come away with fresh ideas -

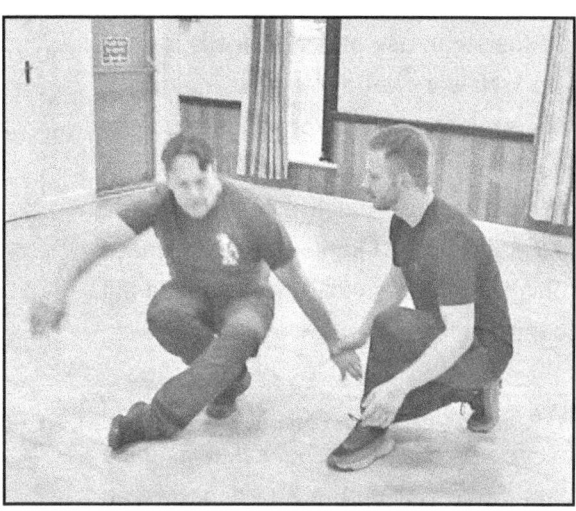

even on subjects I thought I knew a lot about.

That aside, what do we mean by refinement, and what would be an example of how to teach? Let's imagine you were a trainee carpenter, and your job is to make a table. That's easy, right? Four legs, whack a board across them, bang some nails in, *Voilà*, we have a table!

Yes it is, technically and perhaps functionally a table, but it might wobble, it might have nails sticking out, perhaps the surface is rough and gives splinters. As any craftsperson develops, their work becomes smoother, more functional, more refined.

Now, in some ways that is not a great analogy, as with furniture people prize the look of the thing as much as the function. Yet, having said that, there is a joy and appreciation in seeing a person move well, with poise, precision and controlled power, so I'm sticking with it! I think that functionality brings its own aesthetic with it, think of a machine like a Spitfire fighter plane, for example. It's a warplane, it's designed for a specific function. Yet that functionality brought a clearness and flow of design that we can appreciate aesthetically too

In Systema, our prime goal is refinement of function, which usually means getting more by doing less. Let's use a simple takedown as an example.

A stands next to B and places one hand on the head, one on the hip. A tilts B's head back and pushes down, while keeping B's hip in place. B should fall.

The first time people try this, it's not uncommon for A to put a lot of tension into the pushing hand. They try and force B's head back and down, which tends to aggravate B, and lead to the tensing up themselves. The pair then become locked in a tension struggle, where the technique might eventually work, but not without a lot of grunting and pushing - not to mention the risk of injury. So the function is poor, and people may see this as a bad technique.

This is where the instructor steps in and starts showing refinements. The first might be to talk about balance. We all have a balance base, pushing into this does nothing to break balance. So the head needs to be moved out from that base. We might also mention the idea of triangulation in balance. Draw a triangle, the line between the two feet is the base, the apex is the weakest point of balance. Move the heard towards that, and the body will follow.

When that is done, B will naturally step back with a foot to reset the triangle. This is why A checks the hip, to prevent that step from happening. Also, it helps to push in a little on the hip too, just a touch, on order to help break the structure.

Also apply our 3D work from earlier. Don't just take the head back, turn it a little to the side too and press down. Linear force is easily opposed by the body, spiral force less so.

Already, we should have a much more efficient and effective takedown that relies less on tension and more on position. This makes it more effective because when work is applied in a relaxed way, the opponent has less chance of feeling and responding to our movements. But this is still fairly base level. We can work deeper still.

For those first refinements we are looking at what we do to the other person. The next level is to look at what we are doing ourselves. The first thing is our touch - is it light and sensitive, or is it like a bull in a china shop? How do we bring the hands into position - could our movement be made less obvious? Sliding the hand up the back, for example, rather than approaching at eye level?

We should check our own posture and stance. If you feet are widely splayed and we are leaning over, this will not only make our takedown less effective, it will leave us open to counters. So, feet close together, shoulders and hips level.

Now think about how we apply our movement. There is no need for tension in the arms. Once we have decent contact on our target points, simply squat and transfer that movement into the hands. This will apply enough power to do the job. Remember, power is generated through our movement, not by applying tension.

But this is still all outside, or external. We should also be aware of our internal state. How is our breathing, our pulse rate, our psychological as well as physical posture? Systema places a lot of emphasis on being "comfortable" in what we do. We are not working from a position of struggle, but try a much as we can to work from the most comfortable and advantageous place we can, whatever the outside conditions may be. It's an important point to reinforce for students, some of whom may naturally assume that tension and exertion is the key to everything.

As we know, breathing is the best way to help monitor and regulate the internal state, so never be shy in reminding people to breathe as they work! *Place the hands, exhale, sink and turn…*

Take these principles and apply them across all of the work. Not only will this give you several more months of class content, it will ensure your students will develop quickly out of the basics. In fact, I'd go as far to say that with this approach, students develop applicable skills and attributes far quicker than many other methods - mostly because the training works on a behavioural level, rather than on rote learning and repetition.

There is already a lot here, but the next stage is to start working on more of an internal level. This is somewhat of a loaded term in some martial arts circles, and leads to claims of almost supernatural powers and the corresponding mockery of "qi-balls" and delusional masters.

My own definition of internal is simply working with consideration of the internal aspects of the body - the breathing, tension levels, internal structures on the physical level, the psyche, mindset and emotions on the mental level. This covers a huge range of work, including understanding natural movement, developing power, verbal and non verbal communication, managing fear, and so on. In other words, the training now moves to what I consider the professional level. We are beyond someone wanting to play *Greensleeves* on a recorder, into being a "proper" musician!

Again, this is something you need to be experiencing yourself before teaching. It's only been the last few years that I've felt more comfortable teaching certain aspects of internal power, for example, and even then I feel I'm only scratching the surface.

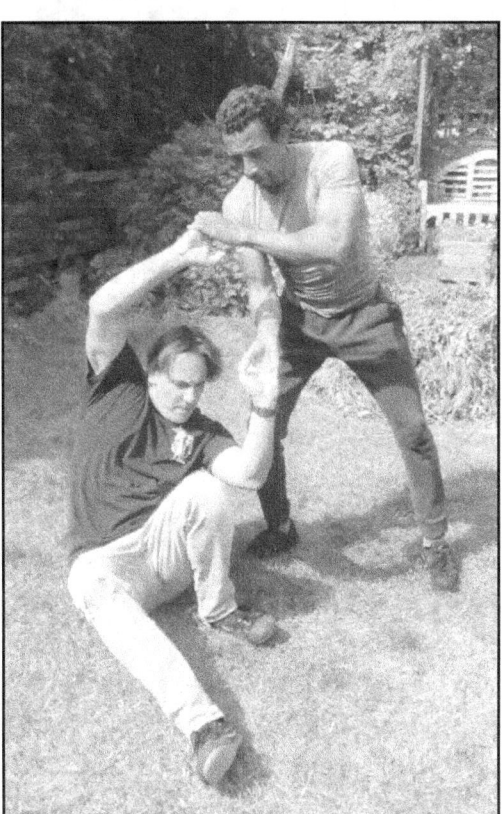

One other thing to mention here, is that you may find resistance from some students when you go to teach more refined work. This is something that caught me by surprise in the early days. I had been teaching primarily from Vladimir's videos and also personal training with him, then went on my first trip to Moscow. I was exposed to some different types of work there that, frankly, blew my mind. Anyway, on my return, I attempted to bring some of those aspects into the regular class.

I quickly found out that some of the students, though by no means all, were happy to come along each week and do the pad work, the push ups, have a bit of a spar, and that was it. They didn't take at all to the refinement work, in fact they left shortly after.

So you may face a decision as an instructor. Stick to what people like, go with the flow, keep things at one level. Or

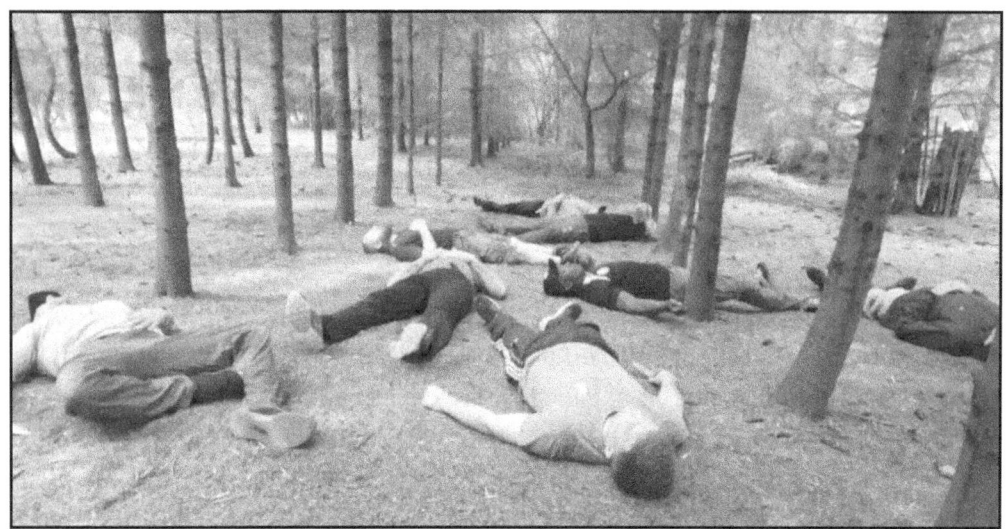

add in more refined work and risk losing people. For me it was no choice, as the more refined work is where I wanted to be going, so that was what we were doing. And still are, or attempting to! And now I have people who fully appreciate that level of training, in fact some say it is what distinguishes our type of training the most from what they have done before.

It is an interesting situation. It never arose in the same way when I started in the traditional styles. There it was made quite clear that "advanced" work was for senior students only. You had to prove your commitment and loyalty to the style (usually by spending a lot of money!) In order to get into that circle. This led to a class dynamic that was great for the ego (if you were one of the chosen few) but which I found unhealthy. And even then, there was still the "secret stuff" that was only revealed to family members or disciples. In short, you never really knew what you were getting, but always had the feeling it wasn't quite everything.

That's another reason I found Systema a breath of fresh air. I've never seen so much as a hint of that attitude. If you want it and train for it, you'll get it. Money aside, I always felt that the whole "secrets" thing was largely self-selective, anyway. Without doing all the hard work, no-one is capable of pulling off the "secrets" anyway. And as I later found out, some of those "secrets" are really quite basic aspects of training that were being deliberately left out of the syllabus.

In that sense, then, students will regulate themselves and their progress. Some will come once a month, some twice a week, some twice a year! Some want a good workout and a bit of punching, others are interested in fight psychology, how to deal with people on physical and non-physical levels, perhaps for their work.

Some prefer a more gentle class, with breathing and movement, though even these can be intense when working at deeper levels. As instructors, we have to recognise all of this and, to some extent, cater for all. Do be aware though, that it is you that sets the tone and pace of the class. If your primary focus is on professional work for door staff, then you might point a person looking only for relaxation and breath work to either one of your other classes, or to another school. That's not to say you can't blend everyone in together, this is usually what happens at our camps or workshops, but those are outside of our general class work.

TESTING

I've mentioned a few times the parallels between how we train in Systema and how people train to become musicians, athletes, and so on. However, musicians get to play live and athletes get to compete. So how do we go about assessing our progress in Systema? Do we even need to? That depends very much on our reasons and motives for training and the personal goals we set for ourselves.

This is where it helps to be clear what your class is about and of what your students are looking for. However, whatever the reasons for both, it is quite straightforward to set up methods of testing.

Let's say you are running a health class. It might be that people come to you with a particular issue. For example, I had one lady with blood pressure problems. After a few months of training, her blood pressure dropped back to normal and she was able (under medical advice) to come off of her medication. Now I know that is not a "test" as such, but it is a measurable effect of training.

For other people, it may be the fact that they can get to do a full push up, or have more general mobility in their day to day life. In fact, often it's day to day life that provides the tests! I mentioned before that one of our senior ladies tripped over recently and, thanks to her falls training, escaped unscathed.

Similar "tests" may be remaining calm in difficult situations, coping better with general stress, not getting out of breath when going up the stairs and so on.

These sort of things apply across the board, but what about our self defence / martial art / professional type work specifically? How can we be sure that what we are training is in practical , is effective in real life? After on, in training we work with partners who don't really want to hurt us, who may not really be trying to stop us doing something, who may be quite compliant. Martial arts are generally tested in four ways: gradings, competition, pressure testing and real life!

Gradings

If you mention that you do martial arts, one of the first questions you will likely be asked is "are you a black belt?" The grading system became a very strong feature of the Japanese arts, and in the public mind is applied to all styles.

In the traditional Chinese styles I came up in, there was generally no grading. Some schools did introduce a sash or belt system later on, but, by and large, there were no gradings, so it is not something I have experience of. I was awarded a black belt 1st dan in a Jujitsu style at one point, though this was because the instructor didn't feel I should be teaching his students without one. Fair enough, his school, his rules.

Gradings are typically done by testing a student's knowledge and ability in the particular syllabus. In stands to reason, then, that gradings work best in a very structured, syllabus driven approach. In other word, you learn certain movements or techniques as you go up the grades.

Could we apply this to Systema? On one level, perhaps. We could test a student's ability to roll well, to perform some lock escapes, or various types of drill and so on. The difficulty comes in applying a "level" to each of these. Take a knife drill - if the knife is avoided and the attacker neutralised, then I guess that is a pass. But could it have been done better?What criteria do we apply? And to what purpose?

We spoke before about internal and external motivations. It may be there is a particular group who would respond well to such testing. However, my experience is that many students have been through that process already and are glad to be away from it. Some see it as too rigid, some as not particularly meaningful, some as basically an excuse to charge the student for gradings, belts, certificates and so on.

In that sense, then, I feel that gradings in Systema are down to the individual instructor, though I don't know of any who use them for anything other than children's classes.

Competition

Competing is an excellent way to test various skill sets. Of course, that is largely

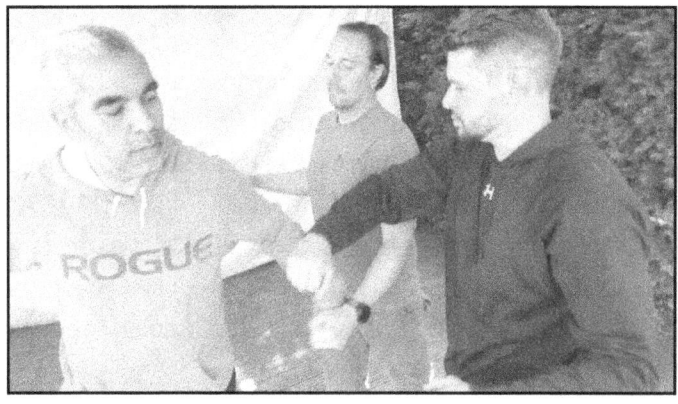

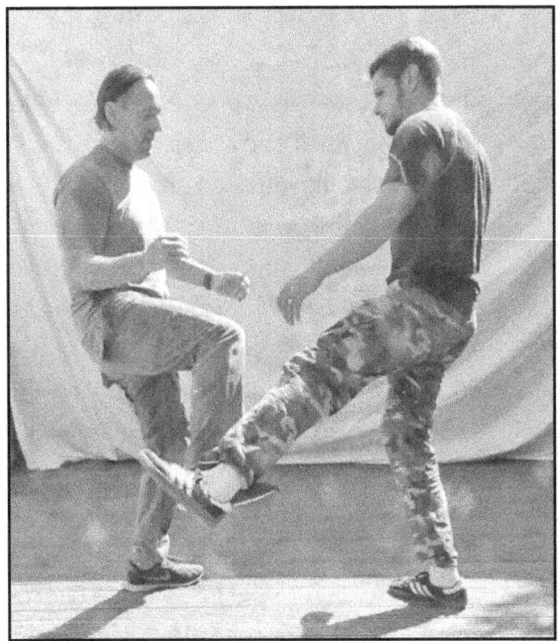

of "real" fighting without the attendant dangers of getting into street fights.

Some of my students are former competitors with no real further interest in it, but I had one lad keen to get into local competitions pre-pandemic, and was looking forward to seeing how we could adapt the training to best help him. I did offer one caveat though - don't get too emotionally involved in the process. A few years back we had a guy who sometimes trained with our group, and got heavily into competing. He dependent on the rule set, but even just was very successful for his first fights, but the pressure of competing can be good when he did eventually lose, it shook him test of how we manage stress. very badly. So keep things in perspective.

Some might be surprised to hear me say that. Sports vs street is one of those tired old arguments that gets trotted out on social media a lot. The polarised extremes are "what we do is too dangerous for sports" and "none your stuff works in the ring, that's why you don't do it."

Thing is, good movement and delivery is good movement and delivery. Granted, there are forbidden techniques for safety, but one aspect of Systema is learning to work within any type of restriction. Competing, then, can be a useful test, particularly for the less experienced person. It will give them some experience

To be honest I'm not a fan of much of the combat sports around at the moment, I feel there has been a huge amount of hype brought in, I find it difficult to watch even the weigh-ins now. Is this really the example we want to set to young people?

That aside, a little healthy competition can be a positive thing, if treated, win or lose, as a learning experience.

Real Life

The ultimate test, we might say, is being in an actual situations. After all, this is what we train for. That situation might be any number of things, from an argument at work to someone trying to shoot you, and everything in-between. I mentioned before about people bringing those experiences back into the class for us to discuss and analyse, in that way the "testing" gets shared among the whole group. Don't neglect this.

But these are events that may just happen, or we wander into. If we really wish to test our capabilities, should we actively be putting ourselves into these situations? That's for the individual to decide. Personally, at the age I'm at now, I'd advise against it. However, when I was a younger man it was, shall we say, not uncommon to be involved in certain types of activity that often led to trouble.

Let's put it this way - we've all watched *Fight Club* and can, perhaps, appreciate the idea of going toe to toe with someone in a safe setting. But this is really competing, with the best will in the world it is still not fully the same as being in a totally open-ended situation. Nothing is, even the best simulation is still a simulation.

It's the easiest thing in the world to start a fight. Go into a pub and knock someone's drink over. Slap a passerby round the back of the head. You'll get into a fight alright, but is this a good test? It is if you don't mind the consequences, which could see you in hospital, in prison or in the morgue. Not advisable, then.

There are, however, jobs which will certainly increase your chances of dealing with conflict. The easiest one to get into is door work / security. I say easiest, these days in the UK at least, you need an SIA badge, not something that was an issue back in the 1980s. At that time I did a little door work around East London, usually working clubs where a friend was DJ-ing. It was a good education for me, partly from the physical angle, but also very much just learning how to deal with people. In a typical night we would get people who were friendly, sarcastic, sober, drunk, bellicose, violent, being sick, didn't want to leave the club and so on - and that might all be one person!

So if you did want to put yourself in a place where you will be tested across the board, from people skills to hands-on, then think about door work. Do your research beforehand, be aware of the costs and consequences (I doubt it is good pay and you will be working late nights) and also be

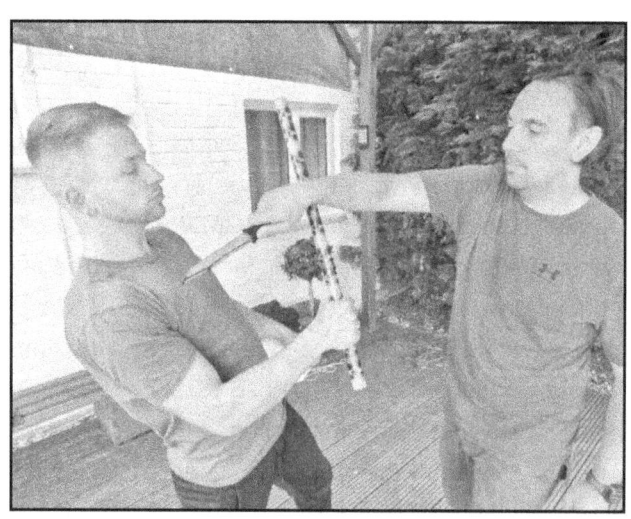

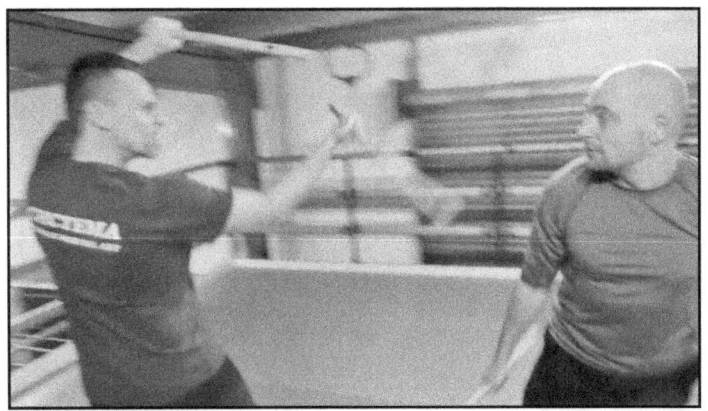

In *Systema Self Defence* I go into detail about how to setup tests and scenarios, but I shall recap the major points here, particularly from an instructor's perspective.

Think back to our section on creating a drill. Pressure Testing is largely the same process, with the main emphasis being the skill or attribute being tested. If we want to test knife defence, then there's little point in running a drill without a knife, for example.

aware of some of the shadier sides of life you might encountered (the drugs trade in particular).

There are other occupations where you will be put to the test - law enforcement springs immediately to mind. However, at least here the UK, they are very set in their ways and procedures which you will have work within. My cousin was a serving police officer a few years back and I showed her some things. She later used on of those to successfully pin and restrain a large, male suspect. She got told off for using a "non-approved technique," even though it worked perfectly and without harm to the suspect. On the other hand, you will have more than ample opportunity to test your people skills and your stress management methods!

Pressure Testing
This is my preferred method for testing, and is easily adaptable for all levels and skill sets.

The next thing is to have some method of determining levels of success or ability in the drill. We can either do this through some form of measurement or by assigning a specific task. For measurement, we might count how many times a person is touched with the knife during the drill. We might even use the white t-shirt and maker pen method for increased clarity.

For task, we give a goal, such as, "you have to restrain your partner within 30 seconds." This way there is not only a clear goal, there is a clear end to the test, too. I mean , this is the case with most exams, right?

Once we have our purpose and criteria for success or failure, we set the framework of the test. How many people are involved, what are their tasks, we can use the Ten

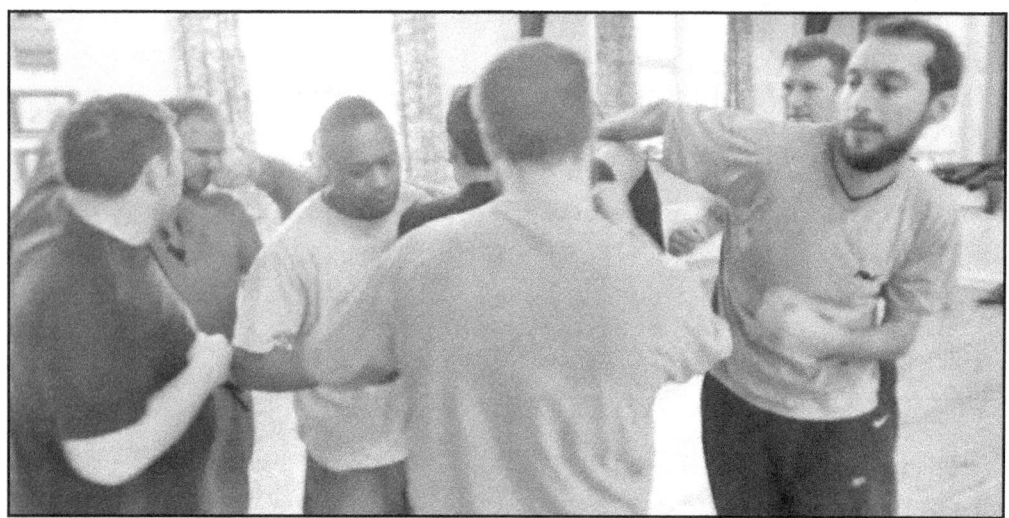

Points template to determine levels of contact, speed and so on. Ensure that everyone is very clear on the test parameters. It is also a good idea to give a safe word in place when testing. If a person says this, the drill ends immediately. This is very important for some of the more intense testing work.

So, we have the test structure in place, along with any equipment required. As an instructor, you know have to think how you will manage the test - what are the stop and start signals, for example. Also, can you monitor the drill and move in to intervene easily if required?

It takes some focus to monitor 20 pairs of people hard sparring - unless you and they are highly experienced. In such a case, it might be better to have, say, three pairs spar at a time, or to delegate watching some pairs to a trusted assistant.

That brings up another issue. I tend to film a fair amount of our class work, for reference, for Youtube and for downloads.

When it comes to testing, I tend not to film as much, and when I do, it is always with the permission of those involved. This is for a couple of reasons.

First, testing can be quite a personal thing. The addition of a camera can have an influence on how people behave, for better or worse. In testing, particularly the more intense drills, we want to see the real person in all their honesty, not an image they might be projecting for social media.

The second is the way such work can be views and judged by outsiders. That, like so many things on social media, is a lose-lose situation. I recently watched one Youtuber criticise Systema for "lack of contact and sparring," then react in genuine horror at people actually getting punched!

There was another gent who proclaims on his channel that "actually hitting each other in training is way too dangerous." So we can't win! I've often said that Systema is both too soft and too hard. Some call out the soft work as "woo-woo" then balk at the fact that we don't use rubber knives.

The other aspect of this is the so-called "break down" or commentaries that we now see. This is where people replay something in slo-mo with attendant critique. It's okay to some extent, I suppose, but isn't it better to be actually doing and showing rather than armchair quarterbacking? Plus I've seen some quite hilarious interpretations of what is actually going on, not just in Systema, I might add.

My favourite Systema one is a young guy commentating on some work in Moscow. At one point, Mikhail picked someone up to adjust their back, which our commentator took as some sort of weird self defence move, with attendant mocking. You have to laugh....

The rise of social media, Youtube in particular, has also encouraged this idea of everything being for your entertainment One of the most distasteful examples of this was the "bum fights" from a while back, where someone would pay two tramps to have a fight, film it and upload it for all to laugh at. That's an extreme example but I do feel it basically boils down to watching two people try and smash each other up for our entertainment. Fair play, some have made a huge industry out of it, though at least professional fighters are there by choice and are getting a cut of the action.

So, we need to be aware when uploading anything of why we are doing it. Are we secretly hoping to "impress" people, or are we just genuinely presenting the work? Something to be aware of.

Back to our testing! Once you have run the test, for however many times you deem necessary, it's good have a post-drill assessment. Ask the people how they think they did, ask observers what they thought. This is where critique is good, it comes from our peers, and from a positive place of understanding. You might want to re-run the drill after this and/or add in any

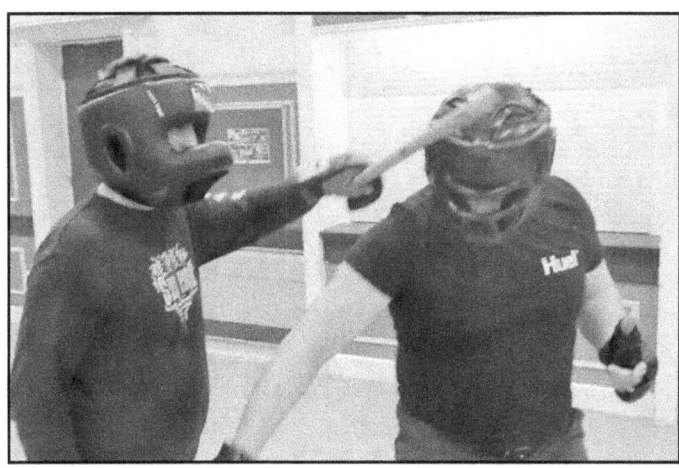

tweaks or variations. You may find that the drill is too much of a challenge, or not enough. In each case you can easily adjust those "faders."

Don't think that this type of testing has to be purely physical, by the way. We can put someone under intense psychological pressure using shouting, slaps, forced breath holds and similar. Again, put a time limit on the drill and make it clear that the aim for the person is to endure the experience while maintaining calm, not to fight their way out. Let's end this chapter by looking at some of the different types of testing drill you can set up.

Solo Task
Could be a breath hold for a certain time, a set number of exercises, getting up and down to the floor without using hands and so on.

Group Task, non-combative
To test movement, have a person go through a gauntlet of sticks, count the number of times they are touched. Or try a team work task, eg the group has to move an "injured" person A from place to place, through obstacles, etc.

Technical Skill
One partner has to apply a particular technique on another, under varying degrees of pressure.

Goal oriented sparring
One or all participants have a specific goal - for example, A must stay in the room, B must remove A from the room

Free sparring
There is no specific goal other than to continue within the framework of the drill. Can be a good test of control and the psyche as well as technical skills.

Situational Testing
We have our goal as before, though perhaps with a secondary goal. We also give a little more context. Eg, A and B are security staff, who need to restrain C.

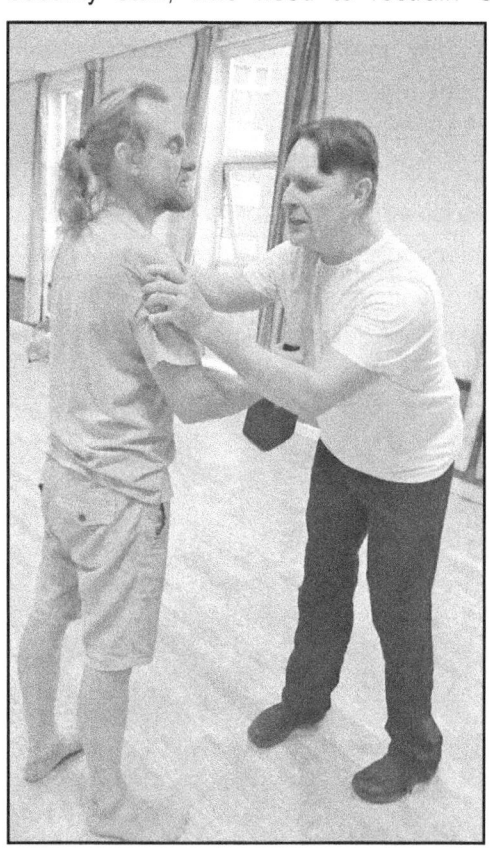

However C is with a group of three friends. Will they intervene or not?

Scenario Testing

This expands on the above into a full simulation of a particular event. If possible, we are in an appropriate location. Let's take our Tuesday night class as an example. Our hall is on the first floor, so we have a flight of stairs to play on (no-one else is in the building at that time.) Prior to this, we will have done some training in fighting and moving on the stairs. From there we could set up a robbery scenario.

For this, everyone is given a specific role and instructions. Hint - not everyone has to know everything. Otherwise it's a bit like peeking at the answer sheet in an exam! It might run something like this.

A - you are on your way home, at the train station. It's late, no-one is around. You take the walkway across to your platform and walk down the steps.

B and C - you've been hanging round the station waiting for an easy mark. You need some cash quickly. Credit cards are okay, but cash is better. One of you has a small folding knife.

D you are walking a few yards behind A, but don't know him. You are on your way home after a long shift at work.

That's the basic set up. You can either instruct people how to act, or let them run with it. So they might be aggressive, friendly, and so on. B and C might "beg" for money, or they may pull the knife straight away.

You then set the limits of the drill in terms of speed, etc. This will largely depend on the abilities of the people involved. The more experienced, the more intense it can be. Once again, the test can be re-run with tweaks applied. We also have to decide what constitutes success in this case. Is losing your money but getting home a win?

Scenarios can be as simple as the previous knife attack scenario, or they can be extremely involved and extend across quite a time. In the past, we have run a scenario drill over a weekend, involving escape, evasion and many other things. This will often depend on time, resources and logistics, but it is possible to run quite extensive scenarios with good preparation and a team of people assisting.

We should also bear in mind that scenario work calls for an element of role play. This can be an issue when everyone knows each other, and even the heaviest verbal aggression can be taken lightly. There is very little you can do about this, except make the situation as real as possible. Try to pair people who don't know each other so well, or use outside people. In the past, we have been able to bring in outsiders, such as a couple of friends of who kindly stepped in as "angry farmers" for one particular exercise. Even though everyone knew we were training, we were able to add a huge amount of uncertainty into the proceedings which certainly added to the experience!

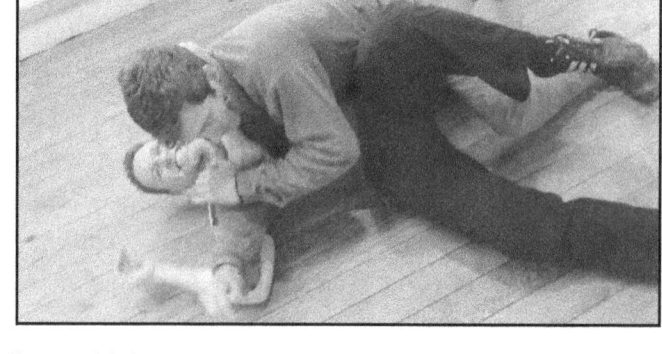

In the usual scenarios we are often calling for a person to be aggressive and intimidating, though this is not always the case. Sometimes we may ask a person to be "procedural" or to act scared or frightened depending on the aims of the drill. Not everyone in the drill has to be an attacker. It may be we have to protect or help someone in difficulty, for example, which then gives us something else to deal with as they hang on to our arm as we work against the attacker!

It is important to point out that there is not necessarily one right way to deal with a particular situation. Running the scenario a few times allows you to explore different approaches and outcomes. It may be best to escape the situation and area, it may be best to ignore the other person, or to calm them down, or to take some direct physical action. Some scenarios are more about surviving the situation and or controlling our fear response than any particular physical action.

It is important that the people taking part understand this. No-one should be under the illusion they are required to be a "tough guy" in every situation. Being low key may be the most important thing, or if you are with family member for example, getting them clear of the trouble zone

At all and every point, always be ready to end a drill or to intervene if required. We spoke about emotions earlier, you can never be quite sure what to expect when people are put under even simulated stress and pressure. If anyone steps out of line, remove them immediately from the training area and calm them down. This has only been necessary twice, in my experience, both under quite intense circumstances. In one case, the student actually went for my fellow instructor - I guess his acting was very good! Still, it was all resolved in the end.

Give some thought to the analysis and de-brief post any testing drill. Do not neglect this!. The longer and more intense the test, the more time for recovery and assessment. Always make sure that people are as stress-free as possible before finishing. I spoke before about those "adrenalise! Adrenalise!" Schools where there is no mechanism given for recovery. Sure, everyone feels stoked - they often even congratulate each other on social media, with a "f–k yeah bro!" For me, I prefer a different approach, but you can experiment as you see fit.

Be careful that testing, and scenarios in particular, don't just become a way for everyone to get hyped up and charge around for a but. I often see in those cases that every technique starts working all the time. This isn't testing, it's bonding. It has its place, perhaps, but is not the purpose of the training, at least not in Systema.

In short, set your test, give each person involved clear instructions, and do a thorough safety assessment, particularly when working outside of the regular class environment. Keep an eye on realism, both in terms of physical capabilities and in terms of consequences, legal and otherwise. Ensure there is a very clear signal to start and end (I usually use a whistle). On hearing the whistle everyone should stop immediately.

Likewise, remember to give people a method of indicating if they wish to leave a drill. They should be free to do so at any point, without judgement. What if is the most common question in martial arts. With Systema we have the opportunity to say, about almost anything, "well, let's give it a try and see…"

CREATING FEAR

We will finish this chapter by looking at some ways to create fear for your students. Pressure is easily created through using the methods already described. Want to make a dill more challenging? Tweak the parameters. Now, that will bring its own type of mental stress as well as physical challenge, but what if we want to work deeper? Are there ways we can put our students into very fearful situations, yet at the same time keep them safe? The answer

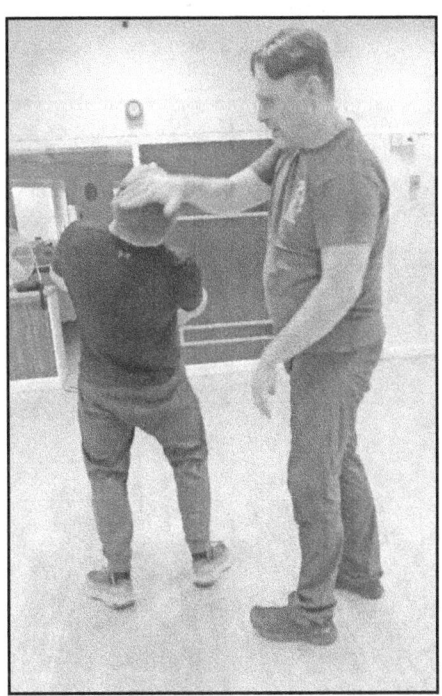

is - yes! With a little thought and a little...misdirection.

I'm going to detail here some of the drills we have used and some I have seen. I'm not going to reveal all the ones we use, as I like to keep some surprises up my sleeve! However, the drills here will give you some ideas from which to develop your own methods.

First, what do we mean by fear? In a training context we are talking about immediate fears rather than existential concerns about the climate, old age, etc. That usually means an over-riding concern for our well-being or physical safety. We might fear walking on a narrow ledge high up, because we don't want to fall and get injured, for example.

Fear is strange, in that it works both off of what we can see and what we can' see! In the case above, I can look down and see the ground way below. However, it also works on what we might think or *imagine* is there. The famed horror writer HP Lovecraft once said "The oldest and strongest emotion of mankind is fear, and the oldest and strongest kind of fear is fear of the unknown."

This tells us that uncertainty breeds fear, that what we don't know can be as scary as what we do know. This is something we can tap into, then, for our drills.

But let's first start with some solo work to help people overcome inhibitors. A universal fear is the fear of falling, so by studying how to fall, we should already be dealing with some issues. Once people have the basics down, you might like to look add in more layers to the work.

I should also state here, in case I haven't made it clear so far - that students should always be provided with the necessary tools to get them through a drill! That is usually a good understanding of breath work and tension/relaxation.

They must know how to regulate and control their psyche before we can test it - otherwise it's like throwing someone into a raging river and expecting them to learn how to swim.

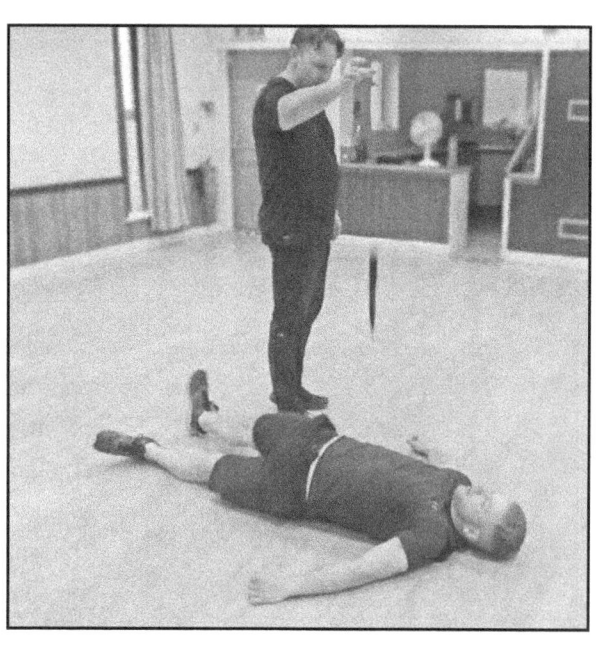

Our first test is to have a person fall forward without using their hands. They start in upright kneeling position, with hands behind the back. The drill is to arch your body forward and to fall on your front, while the hands stay behind the back. A couple of tips - turn the face to the side, and make sure you arch your back in. This forms a curve with the front of your body, so rather than slam into the ground, you kind of rock back and forth on landing. Naturally, it's fine to work on mats at first, but once people have done it, try it on different surfaces.

A very simple move, in one way, but it can be a struggle to overcome that "flinch" challenge to start. As always, inhale, then exhale on the fall. Just do it! I like / don't like this drill as every time I teach it I have to demonstrate! But this is good for an instructor, it stops us getting complacent.

We mentioned the unknown before, and blindfolds are a great way to remove a large swathe of information that we usually rely upon. Even just walking round a familiar room unsighted brings its own challenges. From there, people can move onto falling, being taken down, and even being thrown. Again, ensure each time that students have the requisite falling skills to safely manage the situation.

I spoke about misdirection before, and this is where the blindfold also works well. We set up a situation, blindfold the person, then change the situation without telling them.

The first method is good if you are doing knife-throwing. We first have the person stand (sighted) with their back to the target. The knife thrower aims for the target and the person has to move out of the way. If the thrower is making a big, clear movement, this is not so difficult - though there is an element of fear to start.

After that, we have the person stand against the target, the blindfold is put on, and they are told they have to stand very still. Just prior to the blindfold going on, I make a show of asking someone to bring the First Aid kit out and ready.

The thrower is now going to throw at the target, just like they do in the circus! Except they are not. The thrower mimics the throw, we have a person coming up to the target to stick the knife in by hand with a big *thunk*. Nice and close to the body is best! They move away and we ask the student to remove their blindfold and see just how good a throw it was!

Another option is to use the fear of heights. I actually saw this one used in some army training to good effect. Students are led up to a flat roof or platform, about ten feet up. They are led to the ledge around the roof and told to look over. They are then brought back to the middle, and blindfolded. They are then instructed that they will be led forward to place both feet on the ledge, from

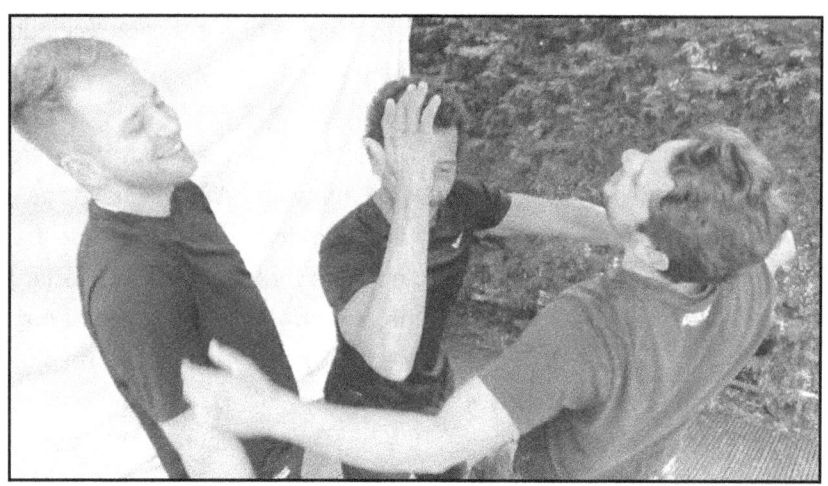

where they must jump (crash mats below are optional!)

Of course, they are not standing on the ledge, they are standing on a bit of wood or similar the same height as the ledge. They are jumping from that to the roof, so a drop of about ten inches rather than ten feet.

This drill can easily be adapted to your environment and, like the forward fall, is a good way of getting people to overcome that flinch reaction. Inhale, exhale, go!

Let's go back to knives, as they bring a lot of fear with them. One we use a lot is the knife drop. A lays on their back. B holds a knife over them. B counts out loud 1-2-3 and drops the knife. A has to avoid it. From there, B counts 1 and drops, then finally makes no sound at all, just drops the knife.

We start this off with a rubber or wooden knife, then progress to training and metal knives. We've run this several times with a live blade without accidents. We usually find that for people used to the drill, the live blade actually improves their response. This is exactly what we are aiming for - people using the fear to assist movement rather than letting it freeze them.

We also adjust the height and position of the knife pre-drop. It makes a big difference if the knife is over your face or your chest, for example. Don't rush into using live blades, and be sensible with what you use. A light knife will likely not do any damage if it does hit - especially if the person is moving well. You may also give the person a thick jacket or similar to wear.

The second knife drill relies on misdirection. Take a sheet of paper and cut if a few times with a sharp knife, in front of the student. Tell them you are going to attack with full out stabs and their job is to avoid contact with the blade. No fighting back, just movement. This is when you switch the live blade for a similar looking training one. I use the "get the first aid kit ready, will you?" moment as a distraction.

If you want to ramp up the fear levels, there are two ways to do it as you set up the drill. The first is to emphasise the risk of injury. That's the purpose for the First Aid kit show.

The second trick is to draw out the situation, to extend as much as you can that period of anticipation - because this is where the fear begins to build. If someone threw a punch at you right now, out of the blue, you'd likely respond in a good way - if you've been training well! However if someone says "I'm coming round tomorrow to beat you up," that creates an anxiety that will be with you all night and into the next day.

Same thing here. Take your time setting the scene. No jokes, put your serious face on and prime others to do the same. Back to our drill. I use the distraction of the First Aid kit coming out to switch knives. Then, when we're set, I go full bore at the student and see how they do.

One last drill. Once again this was blindfold, but you will need a horse! We spent a day training on the farm, including work on and around horses. One of the fear drills was to have students lay on their backs, blindfold, while the horse galloped over them. Of course, the horse was actually nowhere near them, he was happily charging up and down the field twenty feet away! But when you are at ground level, and you *feel* that rumble of hooves.....

One thing to make clear again - all participation is voluntary. People can sit out any drill at any time without judgement. However, with these surprise drills, I ask that they leave the room, otherwise they get to see the trick and so miss out on the chance to experience it later. I also tell people not to write or talk about these drills - one keen student once detailed all this type of work we did at camp on his blog! I asked him to remove it and he did. Why deprive others of the same experience? You can also see why this type of training doesn't go up on Youtube - not only from the surprise perspective but also because some of it might be misconstrued as dangerous, or even bullying and so on.

With a little thought and research you will find many other ways to create fear for your students, yet keep them safe. The main principle is to create either a visually difficult situation or to bring in enough uncertainty to make the student almost forget that it is training and there is a real risk of injury.

When doing blindfold work, be sure to have enough sighted people to intervene if required, and, as with all testing, make sure to provide enough downtime after the drill for discussion and cool down. And if you come up with some good drills, let me know!

CHAPTER NINE
WORKSHOPS

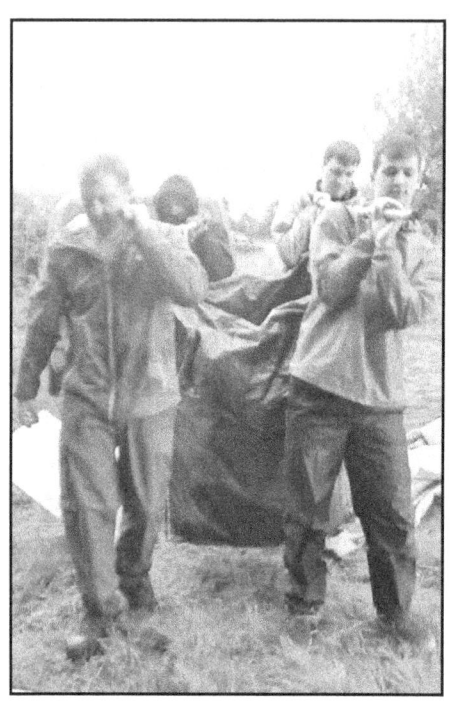

So far we have mostly spoken about regular classes at your usual venue. But we can teach in many other places too, most typically in workshops, courses and camps. The first two might be arranged by yourself, you might be invited to teach a workshop at another club or organisation, or you might be arranging a workshop for a visiting teacher.

Camps are longer events which involve the participants staying over on site. That may be an outdoor camping site, or it might be at a conference venue or similar. Both situations come with some special considerations we must be aware of in addition to those already discussed. Let's start with the easiest, the workshop held for you own students.

IN-HOUSE WORKSHOP

Time in class is always limited, so it is good to have the opportunity to go a little more in-depth on a particular topic. This type of workshop also works well for testing sessions, as they give more time to set up drills and scenarios. If you run a few classes, these workshops are also good opportunities for all your students to gather and train with new and old friends.

All the points pertaining to setting up a class apply here. Your choice of venue, time, etc. Most often I will use one of our regular class venues for this type of workshop - people are familiar with it. The only difference may be if more space is required, or we are working specifically outside, etc.

Once you have your venue, think about the time. How long do you want to be teaching for? Personally, I would expect a minimum of three hours for a workshop, up to six hours. Then you can set your start and end times and date. Be aware of when most people will be around - so usually a weekend, or perhaps a weekday evening. When you set your start time, be aware that some people may have to travel, so factor that in.

That may particularly be the case if you run an open workshop. I tend to, and have been lucky enough to have people travel from all over to attend. For that reason it's best to have a venue with good parking facilities and also somewhere near a station, meaning that anyone coming by train can get there, or can be easily picked up.

What is the aim of the workshop? Are you looking to refine a particular skill or attribute? Perhaps a day on knife defence? Or looking to extend time spent on one type of work - a long session on breath work, perhaps? You can just say "let's see what happens on the day" but I've found that people prefer there to be a specific theme to the day, maybe something you don't get the chance to cover so much in regular class.

If you are not so experienced in the topic, don't be afraid to get someone in. I've invited instructors in for grappling work, airsoft / pistol work, control and restraint and various health and healing methods. You might also split the teaching between yourself and another Systema instructor. Back in the day we used to run an annual Systema Meet. Most of the UK instructors would come along with their students and we'd each teach for 45 minutes or so. It did a lot to build up the Systema community here.

So, we have topic, venue, time. Now you need to promote the event. If it is in-house, this is where having a mailing list or social media group works well. Through that you can let all your students know, even the ones who might have missed a few classes. Other than that we have all the channel previously mentioned.

How much should you charge for a workshop? I like to keep prices within reason, but you need to cover your costs and be compensated for your time. Plus you may have to buy in new kit or equipment for some types of training, so factor that in too. It's always good to have an hourly earning rate in mind, then just apply that to whatever situation you are teaching in. Let's say your rate is £30 per hour. For a two hour class, your hall cost is, say, £50, plus £10 in petrol. So you need to take in £120 to cover everything. That would be a dozen students at £10 each.

Price your workshop in the same way. Your hall cost for five hours would be £125, petrol is still £10. Add in your hourly rate, that adds up to £285. That's ten students at £30 for the day, with a bit extra for any kit.

If you stick to this type of formula you'll not go far wrong. Be careful not to under-price, as we mentioned before, and there some who say the more you charge the more people value, but that is up to you.

One other piece of strong advice - as much as you can, get people to book in advance. That might be in cash when they see you, or set up an online payment method. Most everyone knows how to use Paypal or similar now, and no-one thinks anything of pre-booking to see a movie or a show. I learned this the hard way when first setting up workshops. I'd have 20 people say they would come, no-one paid in advance, five would not turn up on the day. That's no fun when you still have to pay out for the hall, even less so when you have to pay a visiting or guest teacher.

As in incentive, you can offer discount to your regulars, early bird booking prices, and so on. But get people to book, even if it is a non-refundable deposit.

How to structure a workshop? It's largely the same principle as with a class. While I tend to teach classes "on the fly" these days, I do write out a list for workshops. This is as much to remind me of salient points and

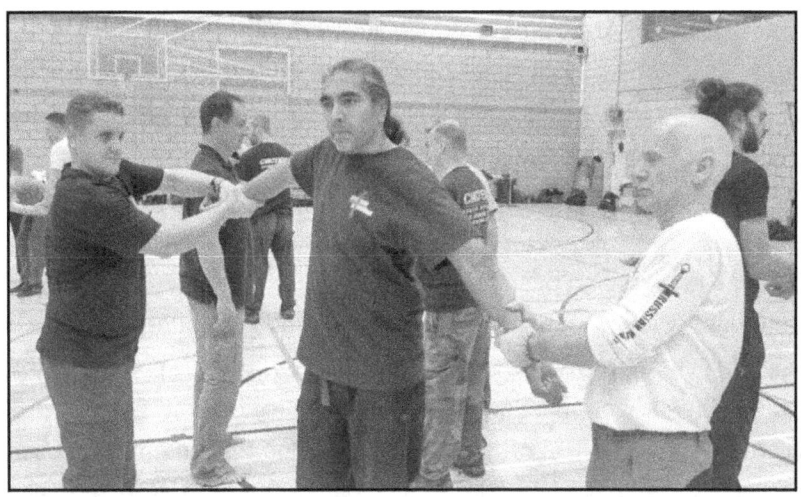

drills as anything, but it also helps give me a structure to work from. Here are my notes, plus some explanation, from a workshop on awareness we ran in 2018. The venue was our usual hall in Tempsford and we had around 15 participants. The workshop ran from 10am to 3pm and the aim of the day was to improve general observation and awareness across a range of situations.

Introduction

General bookkeeping (collect fees, waivers signed if required, point out where facilities are, etc)

Set up diagrams

Hand out pen and paper

Welcome and give brief overview of the day

Explain that "it's all live." In other words, the awareness training for the day is constant. This was to keep students in a permanent state of awareness across the day. One way we did this was to put clear sellotape across certain doorways at eye height. Most saw and avoided, one person walked into it every time!

Explain *indicators*. We are scanning for something new or something missing as a primary indicator of change.

Self Awareness

Basic breathing with selective tension (awareness of internal state)

Pulse breathing - connect breathing with pulse.

Connect breathing with core exercises.

Visual Awareness

Explain vision as our primary sense.

Explain the McGurk effect, where the visual information a person gets from seeing a person speak can change the way they hear the sound.

Eye exercises (rotations, focus, etc)

Explain tunnel and peripheral vision - spotlight and wide beam.

Peripheral or "eagle vision" exercises

Visual drills
Stand opposite partner and copy their movements, large to small. Static and moving.
Partner throws ball from behind over your shoulder - you must catch it. Variations - bounce against wall, throw from under, etc
Partner drops a stick and you must catch it. Vary positions.
Catch a thrown or bounced ball while doing press ups or other exercises.

General Observation drills
Explain commentary method of observation.
Give a minute for people to look around the room. Ask questions, eg what colour are the curtains? How many people are in the room? Memory test - uncover ten objects on a table. Cover again after a minute, people must then list them
Room walk - students walk through a room, in one door, out the other. They are then asked questions eg how many radiators, what colour was the vase on the table, etc.
Blindfold walk - ask people to walk around the perimeter of the hall. Repeat blindfolded.

Observing Others drills
Observe partner, then turn away. They make one change. You tune back and must spot the change. Changes may include posture, putting glasses on, an item of clothing, etc
Ditto except you now observe three people, only one makes a change.
Observe partner, they tense a part of the body - point and vocalise.

Explain body language basic, including stress indicators, postural tells, eye movement indicators.
The Ten Commandments of Observation.
Ask partner three questions, they must lie on one answer, you must guess which it is.

Explain zones of awareness, misdirection, the "spotlight" method
Approach partner "unseen"
Pickpocket principles, blocking, distraction, etc
Pickpocket drills - removing folded paper from pockets, group drill

Tactile Sensitivity
Partners place stick between them and must move without allowing stick to fall
Accept push from stick, move to absorb / redirect it
Basic hand to hand sensing and sticking drills
Explain difference between touch and connection. Using touch to affect structure and balance, static and moving.
Blindfold drills

Combat Applications
Explain OODA loop

BEING A GUEST INSTRUCTOR

Over the years I've taught at numerous multi-style events, been a guest instructor for different clubs and groups, both Systema and other, and taught workplace and corporate seminars. The main thing to remember on these occasions is that you will be teaching "new" people and will be representing not only yourself but the wider Systema community in general. I mention this as one of my first experiences with a guest instructor coming in to my rather new System group was not positive. Fortunately I had already trained with Vladimir, etc so was able to see that situation for what it was.

In other words, we should maintain a professional approach across the whole experience, from start to finish. Sometimes I've had people get in touch with me out of the blue, other times they have been friends who run their own schools who would like their students to experience some Systema.

One of the first questions asked will be "what is your fee?" You can apply the earlier formula to some extent, though bear in mind it will be your host who is now covering all the costs, and it is also fair that they earn something from the event, too.

When guesting you will likely need to travel, you may also need to stay over. How you do that is up to you. If flying, I'm perfectly happy going economy class, and

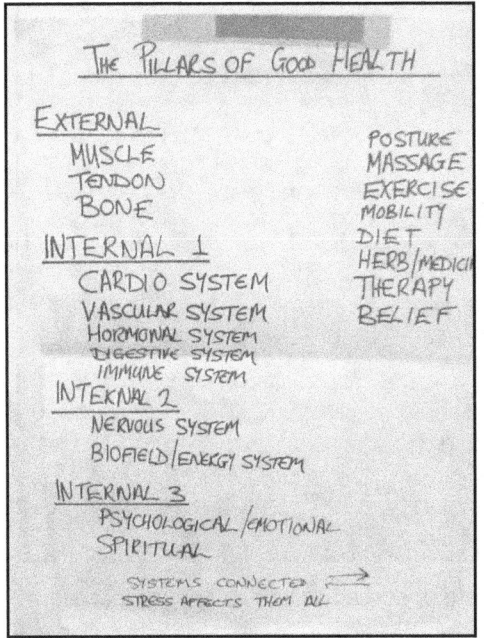

OODA drills - pattern interrupt, cutting into movement, pre-emptive work
Knife spot drills - partner conceals knife, must turn and spot, static and moving.
Repeat with one spotting three (one knife)
.
Add in movements / attacks as required.
Freeform drills / scenarios

Circle and finish
Closing exercises and breathwork
Circle up and finish, feedback and thanks

I mentioned setting up diagrams at the start. I often use these for workshops as handy visual reference fro some of the theory, and also as a good *aide memoire*! I use A2 artist pad sheets and Sharpie pen, pinned up with Blue Tack.

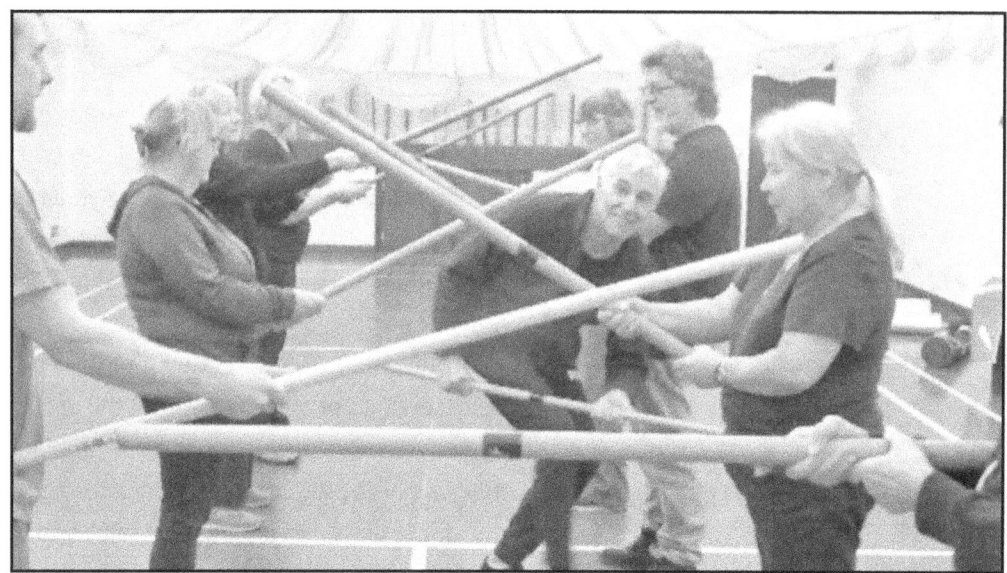

as long as my accommodation has some privacy and a shower, that's fine. You might be tempted to insist on business class and a five star hotel, well that depends on who is inviting you. Factor all those costs into your fee.

It is quite normal to charge more for a corporate client, these generally have a larger budget available, so check around and see what the current market rate is for "expert teachers."

If it is another Systema club, bear in mind the teacher is likely in a similar situation as you - having to pay for halls, advertising and so on, with a group of regular students.

Similar to the hourly rate, I have a set daily rate to hand for such enquiries. This will be adjusted according to the situation. Will you be away from home for a few days, or is the event local? Is your host a mate or someone you've never met before? Check out their website and see what sort of charges they are making for their own school that will give you some guidance, too.

You may find that you are asked to teach at charity events. That is very much up to you, but do be wary. As a musician, charity events are the bane of my life. Bands are constantly asked to perform for free, with the promise that it's "good for exposure." It isn't, and people die of exposure... I also always ask if the sound guy, promoter, bar staff, etc are all getting paid. As well as this, be aware that the more charity events you do, the more you will be known as the "charity guy," happy to work for free.

Be clear on what you are being asked to teach. I'm always happy to teach any aspect of Systema, though I'm more confident with some than others. Again, stick to your lane, don't go teaching sword fighting if you've never picked one up before! Also be clear on times and places There is nothing worse than arriving late when you are a guest. I saw one guest instructor who thought it was fashionable to be late, I guess he thought it would add to his mystique. It didn't, he was never invited back to that particular event,

If it is a multi-style event, be clear on how much time you have for your slot and plan accordingly. Don't over run, you are biting into someone else's time! When you arrive, take some time to chat to the other instructors, don't be aloof. If topics are overlapping, be adaptable. Also, be aware that you are their to teach, not to convert. People have their own styles, these events are to give them a taste of other approaches. Be respectful, don't knock anyone or anything, just present your work clearly and honestly. Don't forget to take any business cards or similar in case people want further details of what you do.

If all that holds for "regular" martial art clubs, then doubly so for workplace or corporate training. Again, be clear on what is expected, be on time, look smart. Also, it is worth checking where exactly you will be teaching. I was booked to do a series of Tai Chi sessions for a local company once. When I got there, it turned out I would be working in an office with all the desks pushed to one side. Not ideal.

Also be aware that corporate clients may ask to see certification, insurance details and so on. Be sure to have something in writing from them, even if it is just an e-mail. Never take any booking over the phone, unless you know the person well. And always feel free to ask for part of your fee up front, particularly if there are extensive travel costs.

One last point is to think about how you are being paid. With corporate clients, you won't be getting cash on the day. Often you will be asked to submit an invoice, and may have to wait some time before being paid.

HOSTING A WORKSHOP

This may a situation where you bring a friend or fellow instructor in to teach, or it may be one of the main teachers from Toronto. Moscow, or elsewhere. If people are travelling a long distance, it will normally be at least a two day workshop. When we first brought Sergei Ozhereliev over, it was for a whole week, so we arranged workshops in London, Cambridge and York for him. It was nice, not only did we get the workshops, we got to show him around the place a bit, too!

In my pre-Systema days I had already hosted teachers from Italy, the USA and China, so it wasn't too much of a reach for me to do the same for Mikhail, Vladimir,

Sergei and Valentin Vasiliev. However if you don't have experience in organising a major event such as these, here are some tips.

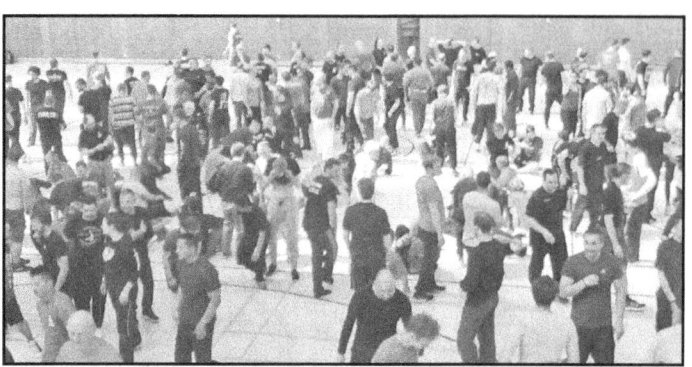

Apply all the same principles as before, only the other way round. Be very clear as to fees, times, dates, venues and so on. On Vladimir's first visit I had an embarrassing mix up between Canadian and US dollars - so be sure to double check everything!

Make sure you have all your expenses outlined up front. That includes instructor fee, cost of accommodation, cost of travel, venue cost, promotion costs. Are you sure you can sell enough tickets to cover everything? Again, be sure to set up an easy way for people to book in advance.

Check what your guest requires in each case. Some instructors may be happy to stay at your house, others may prefer a hotel. One thing - don't haggle! If you find everything is beyond your budget, then be honest and say so. And don't try and cut corners at the expense of your guest, it doesn't go down well. Again, be professional and consider how you would like to be treated in the same situation.

I always maintain that hosting a big event is like hosting a party. You never really enjoy it in the same way you do as if you were a guest. So be prepared to not be so involved in the training, as you will be keeping a eye on everything and everyone and the clock. Be sure to have transport sorted and in place, and a translator if required. Also think about any equipment you might need - much better for people to bring their own if possible. Will you also be supplying bottled water? What about lunch? Will there be an evening meal?

In short, approach it a bit like you are organising a wedding or similar event. Remember, your aim is to provide a good experience for the people and instructors attending, it's about them, not you.

I always liked to video workshops, but check with the guest instructor first. There was once a person who filmed workshops then started selling the tapes without permission, again not a good thing to do. By the way, I normally include in the booking form that filming is not allowed at such events, though taking photos is okay.

One last thing - have some local currency ready to give any instructor visiting from overseas. It allows them to buy a few souvenirs or similar, and makes them feel more welcome.

COURSES

I mentioned corporate workshops above. While I have done some of the those, it is far more common to be asked to run a course, usually in the workplace. As well as our own courses, in the past I have run courses in self defence at a merchant bank, at various colleges, for CPS staff, for RAF Regiment personnel, for youth workers and for PCSOs. I've also run health / fitness courses for teachers at a local school, a large mail order company, office staff and a GP group.

When going into a workplace or similar, all the rules apply as for running a workshop. Be clear, be professional, be focused.

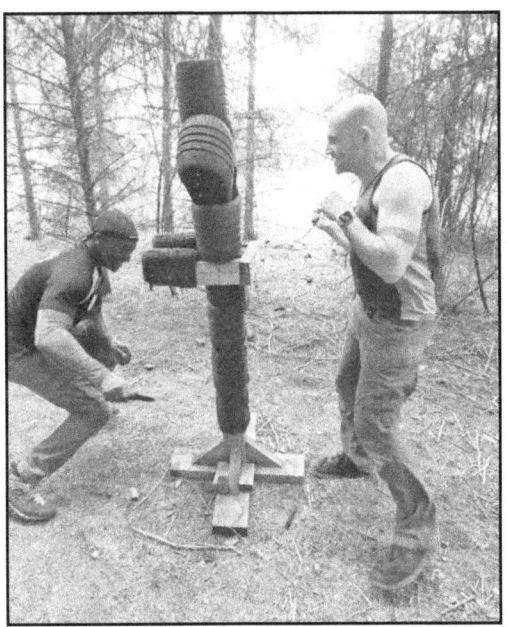

These courses usually take the form of six or so classes. In other words, you have limited time in which to teach. Plan your syllabus accordingly and depending on the needs of the client.

A quick word here about self defence courses. I used to run quite a few of these years back, but far less these days. There are couple of reasons for that. I find that these days there seems little interest in self defence. I'd say from the seventies through to the nineties people were far more interested in it. Maybe things are safer now, maybe people are more concerned with other types of crime.

Also, in many ways I have gone off the idea of teaching "self defence," or at least what most people think of as self defence. I find that people looking for that type of training now tend to gravitate towards Krav Maga, or similar. The mindset for many of them is "show me what to do against an attacker." In other words, they want to learn a few easy moves that will neutralise the baddies and make you look cool while doing so.

My approach to self defence is to first learn how to deal with fear and stress, then to start working on awareness, then look at ways of avoidance and escape. After all that, we might eventually get to practicing some "cool" techniques. The problem is that this approach is not as marketable as the more "dynamic" way. However, it will furnish the average person with a much better set of skills and a strong foundation on which to build their physical skills.

It gets even more ridiculous with knife defence. A while back we had a local group heavily advertising their Knife Defence Day. Yes, in a day they were going to teach absolute newbies how to defend against a knife. I've done something similar myself, though my focus was again on awareness, fear control, seeing how knives are carried and deployed, evasion and first aid. But this day was accompanied by pictures of a lady taking a knife off an attacker, and so on. It was basically teaching a series of rote techniques.

To me this is the equivalent of saying "I'll teach you to play piano in a day." It's obviously nonsense to anyone who understands the complexities involved, but it looks great on a poster. I'm pleased to say their ads drew quite a lot of flack on social media and consequently they had a very low turnout. It's not that we want to put people off learning how to protect themselves and their families, it's that we want to be sure we are giving them the best tools to do so.

Remember my experience with the youth workers workshops? How my approach was exactly what they were looking for, rather than the "kick the knife out of the hand" brigade? I often find this with professional groups. Again, as Vladimir says "professionals see things in a different way." Here's another example.

An ex-military friend of mine was called in to to teach a special forces unit in Canada. He had three days to do so. He told me he spent the first entire morning just on breathwork. At first, he said he could see the confusion and questioning on the faces of the participants. However, very soon they understood the practical worth of what he was teaching and got into the training.

Contrast, again, with the numerous types who have claimed to teach SAS, Navy Seals, etc, in what tend to be very basic "bish bosh bash" methods designed to appeal to the eye. They are usually revealed as fakes in any case.

So if you are asked to teach a self defence course, be aware of the above. Explain to the client your reasons for teaching in the way we do. I usually say something like "the first thing to learn id how to overcome your fear and not freeze. You might know the best move in the world, but if you freeze you can't do anything." Most people will understand, if not, well, they have other options.

To recap, draw up a list of what topics you want to address over the course, and put them together in a logical progression. Read the room when teaching and adjust as you need to. Listen to the concerns of the group, in fact that is a good way to start. That way you can be sure of giving them the skills that are relevant to their situation,

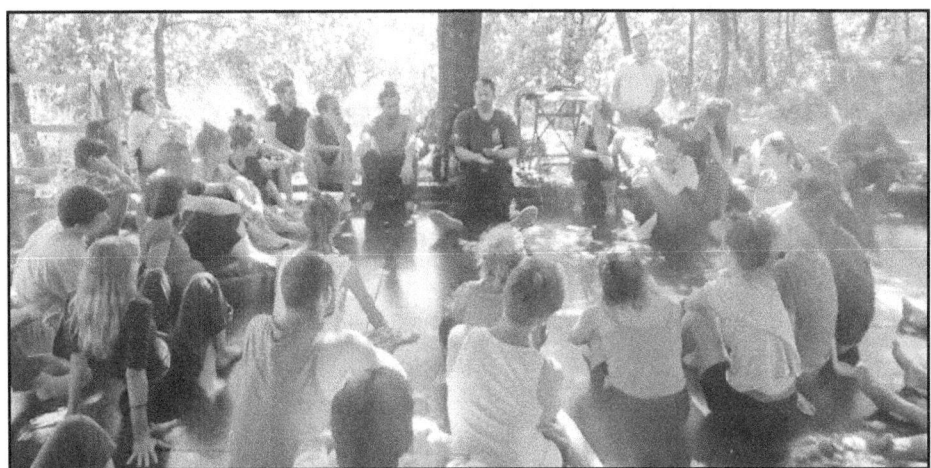

particularly if it is a work environment that carries a risk of physical assault.

If you plan to run your own courses, be they in self defence, fitness, or health, the procedure is the same. What type of person are you appealing to? You might also try running a course as a taster to get people interest in your regular classes., This can work well.

CAMPS

This covers residential workshops, where people are staying over, perhaps for a weekend, perhaps for longer. These give us a great opportunity to dig deeper into the training, as well provide a good social occasion and the chance to try some different work. The best camp I attended as a student was one of the Toronto events, held in a great venue way out in the forests. This was a week of excellent training in field, woods, indoors and water, with excellent facilities, good food and great company. In many ways, this set a template on which we base many of our own events.

The best camp I have been invited to teach at are Bruno and Marina Caverna's Playfight Camps, which were held annually pre-lockdown in Italy. These ran over ten days, with 60 students, in an amazing retreat centre sat atop a large hill overlooking the beautiful Tuscan countryside. The organisation was top notch and I learnt a lot from the experience.

Here in the UK, we've been running annual Systema camps for 17 years, and prior to that, I ran weekend retreats and similar. Once you decide what type of camp you want, the next thing is to find a suitable venue. Here are some of the types that we have used.

Camp site
Official / commercial camp sites
Pros - good facilities, good location

Cons - can be expensive, may restrict your activities, have to bring own food

Wild camping
Public land
Pros - can be secluded and out of the way
Cons - no facilities, public land so dog walkers, etc, some activities may attract attention, have to bring literally everything with you.

Wild camping
Private land
Pros - secluded
Cons - as with other camping, plus it can be difficult getting permission from land owners.

Scout /adventure camps
Private areas set up specifically for outdoor events.
Pros - good facilities, usually have bunk accommodation, a kitchen, etc
Cons - can be expensive, difficult to book as they are usually very busy.

Retreat Centre
These are usually large, old houses that are now set up specifically for weekend retreats.
Pros - excellent facilities, usually provide catering, may have additional features such as spa, etc
Cons - can be costly.

The main consideration for type of venue is what sort of camp or retreat you want it to be. If I were running a health retreat with some more elderly participants, for example, I'd go for the retreat centre, or maybe the scout site. They are unlikely to want to go camping. If it's more of a woodcraft / outdoor oriented event, then camping works well.

Consider which activities you wish to put on and the facilities or equipment you will need to do so. If you want to work stealth and awareness's, it's great to have access to some woodland. If you want to include knife throwing, do you have suitable space and targets? To a large extent, your environment will shape the training.

A word about public and private land, too. Be very sure you know which is which. If you are on private land, be sure you have permission from the relevant person. We have been lucky in that for many years we used a large farm area in Leicester, thanks to the kindness of the owners. That backed on to public land, which was largely woodland, with an old railway track in it that

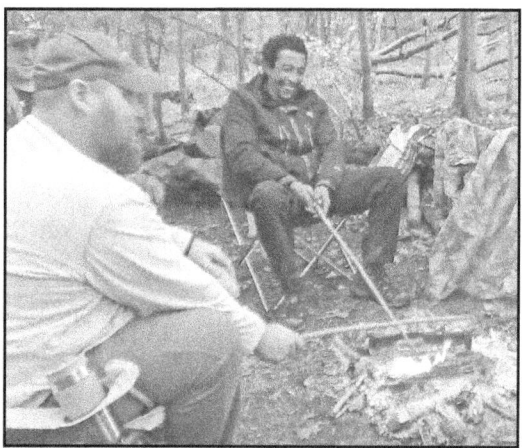

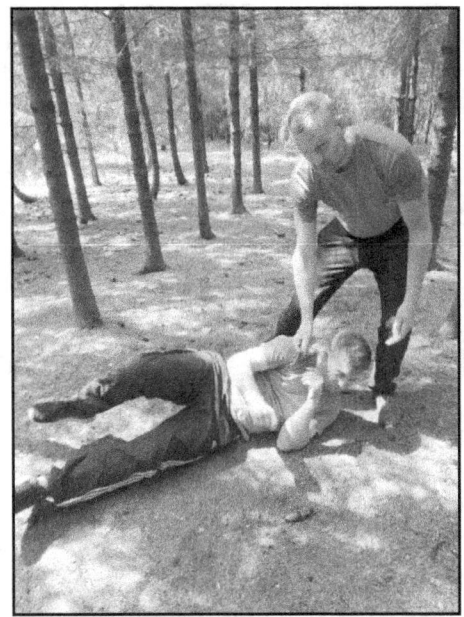

led to an abandoned tunnel. So we were able to use the farm as a base, then train in the woods. The place was very isolated, we never saw another person the whole time we were there.

Another couple of times, we trained in a woodland area that was public. Part of the set up was that participants need to get into the place in an unobtrusive way, so as not to raise concerns from local residents. We managed that a couple of times, then on the third we had a group of participants turn up who decided to hang around chatting loudly at the entrance to the woods, basically being very visible. A complaint went in and the local council investigated. Luckily, by that time we were long gone, but it turns out they didn't approve of people camping in the woods and we were unable to return.

In other cases, we have been in places that we actually knew we weren't supposed to be in. This was an overnight workshop, rather than a camp, which mostly took place in a closed park, that was being patrolled by security. I'm not saying you should do the same, just saying it was an interesting workshop!

Just lately, we have found an excellent place, run by an old neighbour of mine. It is a 37 acre fishing and shooting site, woods, fields and lakes. As I know the owner well, we have no trouble running things like knife work, airsoft, stealth drills, and so on. You may find this more problematic at more public venues. It's understandable, a group of guys dressed in camo gear turning up and knife fighting might cause alarm! So temper your activities with any local concerns.

Personally, I prefer outdoor camps, as I feel this is where Systema really shines. Working in forests really brings out our natural attributes and has an almost instant calming effect on people. The extra time gives us plenty of opportunity to dive deep. But what do you teach, and how?

As usual, look at the time you have to feel, and sketch out a rough program. Lets take a three day woodland camp as an example.

FRIDAY

12pm Site open

Give people time to arrive, to set up their tent, and to settle in.

14.00 - Welcome
Give overview of the weekend, orient people as to facilities / site features. This includes toilets, details of meals, boundaries of the site and so on

H&S - stress any particular safety issues, eg don't go in the river, remember to close all gates and so on.

14.30 Tuning in
We get people to go and sit on their own among the trees and do some quiet breathing.

15.00 Health / Exercise
Stretching, massage, breathwork

16.00 Tea break

16.30 Stick drills
Solo, partner and group. Throw and catch, gauntlets, etc

18.00 Meal break

19.00 Awareness
Range of drills working across al the senses

20.30 Tea Break

21.00 Night training
Team movement, stealth and awareness, low light work

23.30 - campfire

SATURDAY

08.30 Morning Exercise

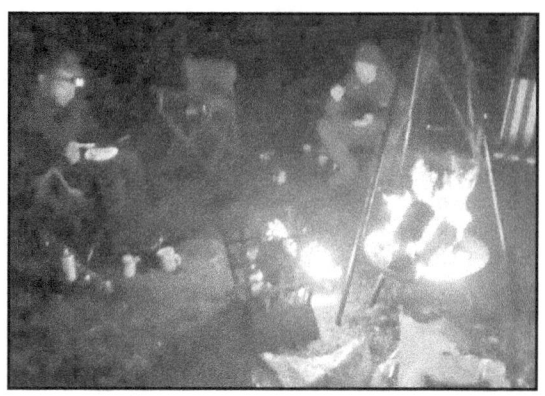

09.00 Breakfast

10.00 Main session
This will be the first session in whatever specialised topic we have decided on . So it might be on knife work, or internal work, etc

12.00 Tea Break

12.30 Exercises / health session

13.30 Meal break

14.30 Main session

16.30 Tea break

17.30 Exercise /health session

18.30 Meal break

19.30 Night training and candle circle

23.30 Campfire

SUNDAY

08.30 Morning Exercise

09.00 Breakfast

10.00 Main session

12.00 Tea Break

12.30 Health / exercise

13.30 Final session

15.00 Closing circle, clear up, pack away and leave.

I know this is short on details, but it is just to provide you with a general framework. It can be tempting to think, right, we will run a series of four hour sessions. This can work for the night training, in fact I would say keep people out in the dark for as long as you can. Not only is there night vision to think about, but also the idea of allowing people time to "sink into" the work and really get into he mindset required.

But outside of that, give people the opportunity to take a break so they can absorb the training, and have a chat and a cup of tea. There is a strong social element to camps. Also, your circle up sessions should be held around the campfire, these are always a highlight of the camps for me.

Just a word on alcohol at camps. Some early camps got quite rowdy, as we had a few people who'd drink heavily on the Friday night. Consequently they weren't in good shape for the morning exercise - in fact one or two even had to go home! So while we all enjoy a few beers, we advise people not to over drink - after all, this is a training camp, not a stag weekend.

The other consideration with a camp is equipment and catering. When people book, I send them a list of required equipment (see Appendices.) So they will need to bring a tent / basha, sleeping bag, etc. You will also need your own, plus you might want a couple of gazebos to use as a kitchen / storage area.

Be clear on what food your are supplying and how you will transport, store and cook it. We generally supply a Friday meal (jacket potatoes can be cooked in advanced and warmed up in a bonfire) and breakfast (fruit, milk, cereals) . Also make sure you have plenty of water available. For cooking, think of bringing in a small gas cooker, or a BBQ or similar. People also enjoy cooking over the fire. Obviously, with any type of fire be very aware of safety issues.

You also need to consider toilet and washing facilities. It might be very basic latrine trench, or you can get portable camping loos quite cheaply now. Be sure there is plenty of hand gel and the like for washing. You also need to plan for things like cutlery, pots and pans, rubbish bags, and so on.

Think also of training equipment. At camp we are more likely to be running activities that need some kit - knife throwing for example, needs knives, targets and frames to hold them up. Think how you are going to transport everything to the site, and also across it. In some places we've had to carry everything in from the cars to deep in the woods. It's best if you can get the whole group involved in this, also in packing the camp away. We have a saying of "leave the place as we found it," there should be no trace that the camp ever took place.

Also, you might need to think about spare kit. It may be that someone forgets something, or maybe their tent gets damaged, or similar. That's all fine, but I remember we once had a person turn up (late) for a camp and literally all he had with him was a six pack of beer in a carrier bag. That was it. He got the same gear list as everyone else, but decided that others would be happy to lend him kit and feed him To be honest, I was all for sending him away, and nowadays I would, but some others leant him spare gear. This is an extreme example, granted, but it can happen!

Incidentally, perhaps with that chap in mind, there is an Appendix on being a good student at the end the book!

I mentioned getting the group involved in packing away earlier. But you should also consider how you want to organise things like booking in, dealing with food and drink, and so on. We have found that what works best is to have a student willing to be in charge of the "kitchen." This might range from simply things like putting the kettle on. Remember, over a small stove, a large kettle might take ages to boil. Better to have someone there to do it, rather than you have to break of teaching to do so. That might range all the way up to actually cooking and preparing and serving food. We are lucky to have a professional chef amongst our number who now deals with all the cooking at camp. It streamlines things and prevents waste.

The large events I mentioned in Tuscany ran along similar lines. Here, a handful of people were offered free or heavily discounted training if they agreed to be helpers. This involved helping out with the food, going off site to get supplies, taking care of equipment and so on. This system also worked very well.

Having said that, also stress that this is a group experience. We like everyone to pitch

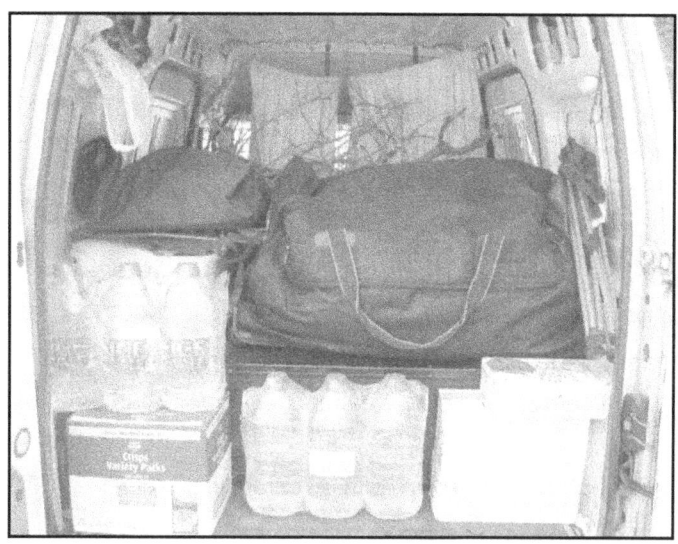

in, bring some food to share and so on. I remember one individual who would do things like wander off during a session to boil a whole kettle and make a cup of tea purely for himself.

We also had one individual who became very disruptive during the campfire circles. Whatever the subject, he was determined to turn it into an argument which really soured the mood on one occasion. Both people were not "invited back" next year. These are rare events but, as with our six-pack friend they can happen and it pays to be prepared.

One very good way to build a good spirit is to run team or partner drills based on cooperation. A little competition can also help. Here's one idea we do for on our Friday night training session .

This is a breathing and sensitivity drill best done in the dark. Split the group into teams of four or five. They stand in a row, with their hands on the shoulder of the person in front. We run them through a series of drills where they have to walk or jog around the area while keeping in synch - that's breath and step. After a while, the team will mesh and start working well as a unit.

Next, have the blindfold except for the one at the rear of the row - this is the driver. Set a course - round the edge of a field, through woods, etc, with a definite start and finish. On the signal, the group moves off. The driver steers by tapping left or right shoulder to turn, pull back to stop. The aim is to complete the circuit as smoothly as possible. Switch drivers each time.

It's easy to pit teams against other, either by timing or by racing at the same time. We find this type of drill is very effective in calming the psyche, increasing sensitivity and really bonding the group together.

INSTRUCTOR WORKSHOPS

The last thing I want to talk about this chapter, are some workshops I have run specifically for instructors. Part of the day was spent covering the issues we have already spoken about, but there were some practical drills and exercises, too. I'll detail them here, so you can try them for yourself. The day was divide into sections, as below.

INTRODUCTION

FIVE W's of teaching - Why? What purpose? Who? Where? When? Promotion, Paperwork (Insurance, disclaimers, etc) Fees and club structure. First aid.

STYLES - Master, coach, fellow student, instructor, Lecture, dictate, lead, teacher feedback. Humour or not?

PRESENTATION
Punctuality and time awareness, appearance, communication skills

Exercises
We then got into our drills, starting with public speaking. To start we run through some basic vocal warm-ups.
Hum your favourite tune.
Run through some scales
Pretend like you're chewing gum. Chew slowly and gently to loosen your jaw.
Swish your tongue around your mouth. Tension sometimes mounts in the back of your tongue and this exercise will loosen and relax it.
Breath control.

Next, each person takes it in turn to address the group. They have to speak for two minutes on a subject of their choice. The group take notes and ask questions at the end of the talk.

Repeat, but this time the speaker is given a topic by one of the group. Two minutes with questions again.

Observe and advise. Point out any problems such as hesitation, "erming", repetition, being nervous, body language, etc.

SETTING UP A CLASS
Linear, modular, freeform teaching. Syllabus, Structure,

Exercise
Write a 90 minute lesson plan from the topics given.

STUDENTS
New students, assessing quickly, determining needs, monitoring/guiding, types of learning.

Exercise
Teach a short drill or exercise to the group for each of the learning types

MANAGING A CLASS
How much to explain? Punctuality, lack of control, disruptive, stop to chat, over-competitive, injury, inappropriate behaviour challenges. You are in charge!

FEEDBACK
During the class – verbal and non-verbal
Circle up

MAKING A DRILL
The Four Pillars for exercise variation.
Ten Points of Sparring for drills.

Exercise
Invent a drill for one of the following - attribute, technical skill, exercise, test, problem solve, psychological - and teach it to the group.

Exercise
One person chooses a topic or sets the goal of a drill. The next person designs the drill,

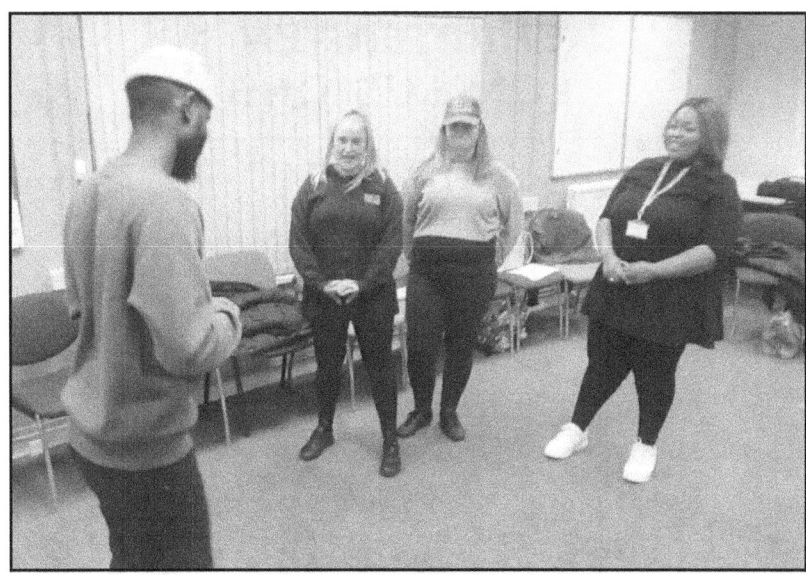

then the next person teaches it to the group.

When a person is teaching you can add in a "difficult student" situation to roleplay. Allow time for feedback after each exercise.

This is the broad outline of each day we ran, and the feedback from participants was very positive. To me, it reinforced the fact that knowing your subject is only half the story. Without half decent communication skills or an amenable personality and presentation, you will likely not be that successful. Teaching is one of those things that looks easy until you try and do it!

Outside of specific training as above, we mostly learn to teach by teaching. So if you have instructors in training in your group, let them take the class for 15 minutes or so - and give them space! Don't hover or make any comment while they are teaching, wait until after the class for suggestions and a debrief.

Alternatively, if you are in a class and have thought about becoming an instructor, the first person to speak to should be you instructor! Follow their guidance, see if they will let you lead the exercises or run some drills under supervision.

Ultimately, you will need to be assessed by Mikhail or Vladimir, of course, if you wish to be a recognised instructor within our school. Should you be successful, then don't forget your old instructor, now it is even more important to keep up your training!

CHAPTER TEN
CONCLUSIONS

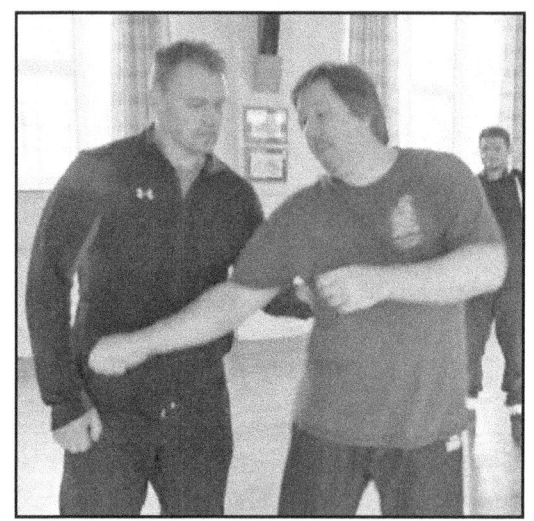

Over the previous chapters we have discussed the many aspects of teaching, from the why, to the where, to the how and beyond. What happens next? How can you develop your classes? Will you grow your school or be happy with a small group? That is all down to you and your skills and motivations. Not everyone is cut out to be an instructor, and I have noticed, over the years, that those who come into teaching for the less positive reasons tend not to be around for long. In fact, I've seen as many come and go as there are still around, maybe more!

It's not a bad idea to think about the future when you first start, as that may also affect how you set your club up. If your plan is build a large school with a string of classes, then start off with your membership structure, etc all in place at the start. It is much easier to do this than try and add things alter on - I've found that people can be quite resistant to change, even in Systema!

Remember, that for most people, this is a hobby. People often look for regularity in their pastimes, otherwise it gets a bit like work! I've seen this happen in some other styles, where the teacher goes from style to style, pinching techniques in order to build their own system. So one month the students are doing Wing Chun punching, the next they are BJJ grappling.

That may be down to genuine "searching" on the part of the instructor, or it may be down to a person trying constantly to pad out a very thin syllabus, or add in more opportunities for expensive gradings. Of course, our own interests may change over time, too, which will be reflected in our teachings.

The reason I first began teaching was to get closer to the teacher and the "advanced" training which was only open to senior students. The club was run like a pyramid scheme - I had to pay my teacher a substantial amount of my earnings, plus sign all my students up as members. I was then expected to bring those students along to workshops at the main school.

This was quite the standard procedure at the time, I guess it still is in many schools. There are other styles who fully adopt the franchise model, with people paying huge amounts of money to be part of the "team."

In other cases, once you get the go ahead to teach, you simply set up your class and go. This may not affect you at first, but think a few years down the line, when you may have students who want to begin teaching. How will you handle that?

I've covered some ideas for class content in this book but, as we know, it would take several huge volumes to list out every single possible training method. I hope that I have given you enough at least for a start, and some templates and methods for developing your own methods. We all start

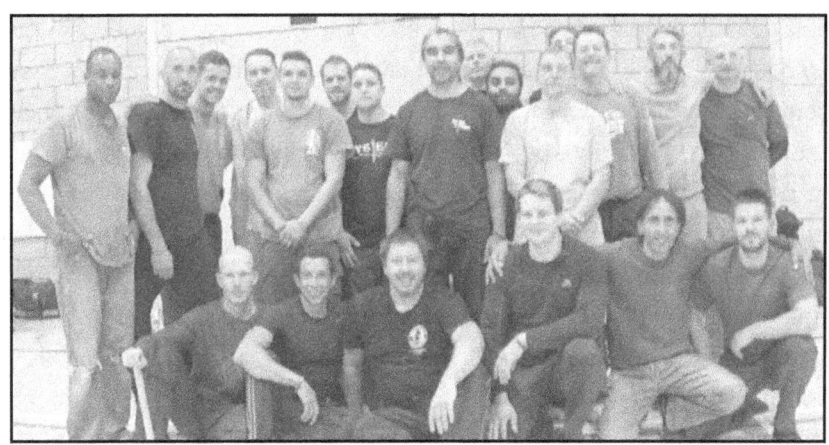

off copying at first, whether that is in martial arts, music or painting. Over time, we develop our own unique style and approach, particularly in Systema, which is more of a living, developing entity than a museum piece. Just always be sure to be working within the core principles and values. If in doubt, you can always check with HQ.

One thing I have not touched on so much here is the heath and well-being aspect of Systema. There are numerous methods built-in, from massage to cold water dousing to fasting, etc. None of these should be neglected in the "martial" side, in fact they are even more important then. Personally, I dislike the distinction between "martial" and "health" training, you tend to get a lot of this separation in some other arts. To me, it is all just training. So please don't feel that your students are "too tough" for massage, or too frail for stick drills.

I found that my senior group love doing stick gauntlets, for example! It's almost as though they become children again, moving round and laughing without a care in the world. This is where the true power of Systema lies, in the transformative effect that it has. Well, perhaps not so much transformative as taking us back to a more natural way of breathing, moving and being. These apparently simple drills have a very strong behavioural impact that will resonate in every aspect of a person's life. It is up to us as instructors, to ensure that this impact is wholly positive (even when it's uncomfortable) and to not shy away from those aspects of training.

I have mentioned before that Mikhail says "people come to you because they need help." Learn to recognise that, and what help it is that people need - not what you think they need, but what they actually need. It may be that you can help them, even if that means just steering them in the right direction. That may be from a physical or mental health issue, it may be from a person at a low ebb in their life, or someone looking to change destructive behavioural patterns.

Don't forget that instructors need help, too! You may find at points that dealing with other people's issues become am issue in itself. This is why it is very important to maintain contact with those further up the line. We not only need to continually implore our own skills, but also to deal with our own issues and shortcomings. It can be easy, if you've had a bad day or are feeling frustrated or angry, to take it out on students. I've seen it happen in other schools. Think back to our idea of the professional mindset and always represent yourself accordingly.

My very first class, teaching on my own, was at a hall in Brentwood, Essex, in the mid 1980s, so I've been teaching martial art for around 35 years. I can still remember how nervous I was at that class, with a group of around a dozen new faces all peering at me. I still cringe at some of the mistakes I've made on the way, but that is all part of the learning process.

Over the years I've tried most types of class set up, from being the instructor for someone else's school, to setting up my own school with two colleagues, to going it alone, to partnering up with a friend to set up our own school and style. I've run quite formal and totally informal classes, with and without memberships, more intense, less intense, combatives based, purely health based. My youngest students have been young kids, the oldest in their mid-80s.

Which is the best approach to take? I can't answer that, it is down to who you are and what type of school you want to run. These days, I personally prefer to keep things low key and generally train a small group from my home or larger groups at workshops. I'm lucky to have been invited to teach all over the UK and Europe, and always look forward to such occasions.

If your first priority is not, above all else, to give your students a positive and educational experience, then please, don't start teaching. If you start from any other base then that, my feeling is you will not do well. Certainly, there are some who have done very well financially out of charging super high fees for little or no actual knowledge, particularly in the heyday of the Kung Fu boom. But I feel those days are largely gone, probably for the best. People today are way more educated with regards to martial arts - though that also has a negative aspect, as we have mentioned with our comments on social media.

In short, be honest and up-front in your teachings, and everything else will fall into place.

Good luck!

APPENDIX ONE

CLASS NOTES

Here's a sample of some class notes ranging over the past few years. They are taken from my old blog and my current Facebook page.
Links are below if you would like to see more.

https://www.facebook.com/groups/CuttingEdgeSystema

http://robpoyton.blogspot.com/

1. Jogging with pyramid breathing, breath holds
2. Core exercises
3. Upper body work with long sticks
4. Free movement with stick
5. Developing joint rotation with stick
6. Deflection / passing vs one and two sticks, slow to fast
7. Ditto vs punches
8. Rotation around point of contact
9. Multiple strikes from initial defensive contact
10. Using partner's shoulder movement as signal to move
11. Blasting forward on the pads
12. DItto on a partner
13. Sword work as the source of punching work - deflect and cut
14. Footwork for positioning, evade into your counter attack
15. Battlefield mentality vs sparring mentality
16. "Invisible" strikes
18. Taking hits and massage
19. Circle up

1. Breathe, stretch, core exercises
2. Pushing with fists in pairs
3. Grab and escape in pairs
4. Allow grab, give support, then disrupt structure with small movement
5. Grab and escape free play

6. Knife from contact -basic movement, left/right up/down
7. Ditto, control the wrist, control the person
8. Quick disarms from contact into control work
9. Vs stabs and slashes - avoid the knife, but make contact with the stabbing arm
10. Ditto in pairs
11. Move and attack the stabbing arm
12. Attack the arm then into the face / body
13. Short work vs the knife
14. The importance of hiding work, legal implications of knife defence
15. Establishing a "day to day " mindset - ie not having a "special mindset" that you have to work from, which needs some preparation time
16. Maintaining physical and psychological equilibrium in training
17. Knife vs knife
18. The elbow is stronger than the chin!
19. Circle and finish

1. Joint rotation and stretching
2. Core exercises
3. Get pushed
4. Pushed to the floor and get up again
5. Get pushed by a group
6. Get slapped around by the group
7. Two vs one - positioning

8. Ditto - work vs legs then the arms
9. Using person as a shield
10. Drop one attacker instantly
11. Guard or no guard?
12. Redirecting strikes
13. Attack the first guy on the way to attacking the second one
14. Taking strikes
15. Relaxing muscles through pressure and massage
16. Circle and finish

1. Stick exercises
2. Assisted squats for knees
3. Stick pushes
4. Stick flow drill
5. Stick locking drill
6. Stick deflection / hit drill
7. Short strike work - drop and catch
8. Fist to fist support - activating tendons
9. Keeping pressure / stress out of the body
10. Power through relaxation
11. Developing power in the hand - the "power bar"
12. Lift fist into push
13. Lift fist into pulse
14. The hand rotation strike, three levels
15. Gauging depth of strike and effect
16. Free sparring
17. Circle and finish

1. Stick warm up
2. Partner stretching with stick
3. Massage with stick
4. Calf walk massage
5. Ladder breath holds and recovery with core exercises
6. Ditto vs pushes and slaps
6. Short stick pushing and taking hits
7. Short stick pad work, basic figure 8
8. Short stick flow hit drill

9. Short strikes with stick
10. Free sparring, punches
11. Massage
12. Circle and finish

1. Stick warm up
2. Power training
3. Pushing with fist, increased resistance
4. Loading from shoulder, elbow, fist
5. Changing angle to break resistance
6. Taking balance on first contact
7. Light touch, sink in, release power
8. Recycling opponent's power, contact and non-contact
9. Application vs punch
10. Free sparring with power application, not flicky flicky
11. Footwork vs sword
12. Avoid and respond, with power
13. Free sword sparring
14. Partner core exercises
15. Circle and finish

1. Floor work - breathing and stretching
2. Isolated movement and rolling
3. Seated position and knee walking
4. Evading kicks and stamps
5. Defending kicks and stamps
6. Pushups with kicks
7. Standing work - pushing with fist
8. Neutralising push
9. Internal support, not rooting into legs
10. Ditto vs strikes
11. Take and return strikes
12. Working to the body - position of fist on ribs
13. Pushing from this position
14. Getting into position, first method - two high strikes to body shot
15. Variations
16. Circle and finish
17. Always work with as much freedom as

possible. You have options, don't close yourself off to them

1. Hammer time
2. Stick strength drill
3. Knife work - pushing with blade
4. Flow drill
5. Ditto with minimal movement
6. Ditto full speed
7. Evasion - opening up and large movement
8. Ditto vs three attackers
9. Controlling / dominating space and moving into gaps
10. Working one ahead
11. Evasion - small movement
12. Shielding and "disappearing"
13. Moving into space safely
14. Adapting body shop and close-in work
15. Snare rather than grab work - smoothness and instant control
16. Extended free sparring
17. Live blade work
18. Punch massage
19. Circle and finish
20. Cohesion and adaptability, progressions in training and the therapeutic aspects of flow state

1. Breathing with selective tension
2. Core exercises with breath holds
3. Pushing with fist
4. Grab and escape
5. Grab and push
6. Pad work with breath holds
7. Working with jacket - mobile and static, solo
8. Grabs, escaping from jacket
9. Use of jacket for takedowns
10. Use of belt vs grabs and strikes
11. Use of book, pen, etc
12. Improvised weapon use - pros and cons
13. Be adaptable, not specific
14. Everything is a weapon
15. Circle and finish

Fear Control Workshop Notes

1. Need to control fear rather than be controlled by it
2. Method – inoculation rather than suppression / de-sensitisation
3. Establishing fear hierarchy
4. Triune brain theory, aggression / predator / human
5. Controlling tension through breathing
6. Basic breath hold and restoration
7. Restoration under discomfort
8. The role of the amygdala / hippocampus
9. The physiology of fear
10. Re-programming the brain, establishing a mindset
11. Using the breath to unlock freeze response
12. Pain management through breathing
13. Basic falls
14. Basic strike management
15. Blindfold work
16. Restoration via breathing and massage
17. Overall principle – to establish a mindset which can respond to fear / stress in a rational way, without undue tension and panic. It's not about "toughing things out", it's about working through a series of drills and exercises of different intensity in order to undergo an experience you can learn from.

APPENDIX TWO

WAIVER EXAMPLES

These are the current waivers I use for general classes and for workshops.

CLASS

I declare that to the best of my knowledge, the information given above is correct and that I know of no reason why I should not participate in Systema training. I understand that I enter any training at my own risk and I waive any legal recourse for damages or injuries or deterioration of health which may arise from my participation. I will proceed with caution during the training and will work within my own limits. I shall not hold responsible Cutting Edge Systema, its Instructors or any of my fellow members, for any injury or harm I may sustain. I understand that in circumstances of an existing medical condition, I should seek approval from my GP before undertaking any training. The above information is accurate and if any changes occur I will inform my instructor immediately.

WORKSHOP

To the best of my knowledge, I am in good physical condition and fully able to participate in this workshop. am fully aware of the risks and hazards connected with participation in Systema including physical injury or even death, and hereby elect to voluntarily participate in said event, knowing that the associated physical activity may be hazardous to me and my property.

I VOLUNTARILY ASSUME FULL RESPONSIBILITY FOR ANY RISKS OR LOSS, PROPERTY DAMAGE, OR PERSONAL INJURY, INCLUDING DEATH, that may be sustained by me, or loss or damage to property owned by me, as a result of participation in this workshop. I further certify that I am at least 18 years of age. I hereby RELEASE, WAIVE, DISCHARGE, AND COVENANT NOT TO SUE, Cutting Edge Systema their officers, servants, agents, and employees (hereinafter referred to as RELEASEES) from any and all liability, claims, demands, actions and causes of action whatsoever arising out of or related to any loss, damage, or injury, including death, that may be sustained by me, or to any property belonging to me, while participating in physical activity, or while on or upon the premises where the event is being conducted.

It is my expressed intent that this release and hold harmless agreement shall bind the members of my family and spouse, if I am alive, and my heirs, assigns and personal representative, if I am deceased, and shall be deemed as a RELEASE, WAIVE, DISCHARGE, and CONVENTION TO SUE the above named RELEASEES. I hereby further agree that this Waiver of Liability and Hold Harmless Agreement shall be constructed in accordance with the laws of the UK.

In signing this release, I acknowledge and represent that I HAVE READ THE FOREGOING Waiver of Liability and Hold Harmless Agreement, UNDERSTAND IT AND SIGN IT VOLUNTARILY as my own free act and deed; no oral representations,statements or inducements, apart from the foregoing written agreements have been made; and I EXECUTE THIS RELEASE FOR FULL, ADEQUATE AND COMPLETE CONSIDERATION FULLY INTENDING TO BE BOUND BY SAME.

APPENDIX THREE

THE SEVEN PRINCIPLES OF BREATHING

1. PATHWAY
Inhale through nose; exhale through mouth

2. LEADING
Let breath slightly lead physical action in time

3. SUFFICIENCY
Take as much breath as you need at the moment, for the action, not more not less

4. CONTINUITY
Keep breathing, without interruption or holding, no matter what you are doing unless doing a special breath-hold training)

5. PENDULUM
Let every breath cycle complete itself and reverse naturally, as a pendulum swings and reverses naturally without interference. Allow, and experience, the reversal pause at the end of each cycle

6. INDEPENDENCE
No specific type of action is invariantly tied to any particular phase of breath cycle (i.e. you should be able to punch or roll as well on inhale as exhale)

7. NO TENSION
Keep your muscles and your body overall relaxed.

APPENDIX FOUR

THE NINE REQUIREMENTS FOR FLOW

In one of the largest psychology studies ever conducted, spanning over twenty years, Mihalyi Csikszentimihalyi found that when people felt their best and performed their best they were in a state of 'flow'. Csikszentimihalyi's research found that the flow state experience was comprised of nine key dimensions.

1. Challenge-skills balance
An equal balance between skill level and challenge. If the challenge is too demanding, we get frustrated. If too easy, we get bored. In flow state, we feel engaged, but not overwhelmed.

2. Action-awareness merging
We are often thinking about something that has happened, or might happen. We live in the past or the future. In flow state, we are completely absorbed in the task at hand.

3. Clear Goals
In many situations, there are contradictory demands and it is sometimes unclear what should occupy our attention. However, in flow state, we have a clear purpose and good grasp of what to do next.

4. Unambiguous feedback
Direct and immediate feedback is continuously present so that we are able to constantly adjust our reactions to meet the current demands. In flow state, we know how well we are doing, all the time.

5. Concentration on the task at hand
High levels of concentration narrows our attention and excludes all unnecessary distractions. Because we are absorbed in the activity, we are only aware of what is relevant to the task at hand, and we do not think about unrelated things.

6. Sense of control
An absolute sense of personal control exists, as if we are able to do anything we want to do.

7. Loss of self-consciousness
Self-consciousness disappears. We often spend a lot of mental energy monitoring how we appear to others. In a flow state, we are too involved in the activity to care about protecting our ego.

8. Transformation of time
A distorted sense of time occurs. Time either slows down or flies by when we are completely engaged in the moment.

9. Autotelic experience
Flow is an intrinsically rewarding activity; the activity becomes autotelic, an end in itself, done for its own sake.

APPENDIX FIVE

CAMP INFORMATION EXAMPLE

These are the current waivers I use for general classes and for workshops.

CUTTING EDGE SYSTEMA SUMMER CAMP 2013

LOCATION
The Clophill Centre Shefford Road, Clophill, Beds. MK45 4BT

DIRECTIONS
From A1 exit at J10 onto the A507 and head for Clophill.
After approx 10 min you will see Beadlow Manor on your left. Just past that take the right turn into Shefford Road. Follow Shefford Road round to the left and the Centre entrance is a couple of hundred yards on the right (there will be a Systema sign up).

From M1 Exit at J12 or J13 and get onto the A507. At the Clophill roundabout go straight over and turn into Shefford Road on the left

There is plenty of car parking space on-site

Public Transport
We can arrange pick up from: Bedford station on Friday afternoon
Flitwick or Arlesey station Fri / Sat

The site will be open from 4pm Friday 16th. Estimated finish time is 2pm Sunday 18th

EQUIPMENT
You will need to bring:
Bedding - sleeping bag
Optional - tent or cover if you don't have a tent shared sleeping spaces in the Yurt are available
Training gear - blunt training knife, blindfold, broom handle or similar stick
Clothing - weather appropriate clothing and footwear. Most of the training will be outdoors
Misc - a torch and batteries, plastic bucket, toiletries (shower available on-site), towel, wet wipes, camera (stills only, no video), notebook and pen
Food - a couple of bottles of water / drinks, snacks
Optional - some wood for the fire!

We will provide breakfast each day (porridge, tea, fruit) plus all food for the Saturday night BBQ
If there is anything you want to bring you think will assist training then please do - better to have it and not need it than vice versa!

WORK

The training over the weekend will be built around the theme of Back to Nature - for a couple of days you can "get away from it all" and immerse yourself in the training experience

We aim to give you a good understanding of how to use natural movement and good posture to keep yourself fit and healthy and how these attributes are used in self defence and combat

We will be teaching a range of exercises to develop mobility, strength and power generation, alongside drills to develop attributes such as sensitivity, awareness, psychological strength and free movement

Our camps vary in physical and psychological intensity, this camp is suitable for people with no prior Systema training and, as always, participation in any drill or exercise is optional

CONTACT

Rob Poyton 075*****   (this number can also be used should you need to be contacted over the weekend)

E-mail   poyton@***

If you have any specific dietary or travel requirements please let me know as soon as possible. Feel free to ask if you have any other questions at all

Ed Phillips and I look forward to meeting you and to an enjoyable camp!

APPENDIX SIX

HOW TO BE A GOOD STUDENT

Let's look at the other side of the coin now, with some ideas and advice on how to get the best from your training experience. Let's assume you are joining a totally new class to start with.

First, make sure you have all the information, class time and place, what you need to bring and the cost. When arriving for the class, be punctual. It may be you need to get there a little early, some instructors like to chat with a new student before class begins.

Dress appropriately. There may be a club uniform or particular type of clothing, it may be you are free to wear anything. In that case be sure it is something you will be comfortable training in. Also be aware of the environment – if it is outdoors, dress according to local conditions.

Listen carefully to all instructions given. If you are not sure about anything, ask either the instructor or another student

When training, remain within the boundaries set by the drill, this will help you get the most from it.

Safety – your training partner's safety is your highest priority, you are both there to learn and help each other

Ask! Never be worried about asking a question. But by the same token, take in the answer and use the information. Also be prepared to share your own knowledge with the group

Equipment – if the club is using training gear, it is very useful to get your own. This may be things like a stick, training knife, focus pads and so on. Your own instructor will advise you. This saves the instructor bringing a huge bag of kit to every session and also means if you have equipment to had – you can use it!

Be creative – Systema in particular is about finding your own way to do things, rather than being put into a "style". Some drills are designed specifically for you to be creative and try different things. Don't be afraid to do so and be wary of getting stuck doing everything the same old way. Working like this will open new neural pathways within the body and will help you develop in ways you never thought of!

Develop an analytical mindset – before and after a drill, think about what you are doing, analyse it from different perspectives, think about how you can improve your response

Be honest – we all have limits, we all have fears and tensions, we all have ego. When these things are highlighted, or sometimes "pricked", in training, be honest about it. Don't suppress feelings but allow them to come out and deal with them. Some of the training is designed to make you emotional. Some of it is designed to break down inner tension and resistance. The worst thing to do is to try and "tough things out". This means you will keep all your existing tension, plus that added in by the drill. Think of it like a heavy weight – you want to ditch it, not add to it and carry it around.

Enjoy! Good training should be something that enhances your life. If you constantly come home from training feeling angry, upset, tense or injured I'd suggest there is a problem. See how your training can positively influence other aspects of your life and how you interact with the people around you

APPENDIX SEVEN

WORKSHOP FEEDBACK

From a student following a major workshop.

Yesterday's workshop highlighted some important points for me:

1. How lucky we are to have experienced people in the group who are willing to share their knowledge during a session. This is something that was unheard of in much of my previous styles of training. It wasn't until training with Vladimir and Mikhail (both of whom think nothing of giving the floor to another person to show some technique or illustrate a point) that I really saw this and appreciated it as valuable aspect of teaching.

2. We were also lucky to have visitors / instructors from other schools attend the workshop. This spirit of openness is always encouraging. Our own guys have always been free to train with whomever they want – which is part of the experience they bring back to the group.

3. I always feel grateful that people choose to come and train with our group. There is a lot of choice out there, even in something as "obscure" as Russian martial arts. On a personal level I have limited time and money so have to be very particular about where I train. I'm not interested in training with someone purely because of their nationality or the thought that they might make me an "instructor" or if all they demonstrate is, to be blunt, on the same level as what we are already doing. The idea that I am told who I can and cannot train with is wholly false. Over the past few years I've trained with a number of teachers in and outside of my RMA circles and there are still a couple on my list I'd like to see.

4. I mentioned at the end of the session, I don't think I've ever heard so much laughter in a workshop as yesterday. Humour is a big part of our training and I wouldn't have it any other way. A few people mentioned the concept of "play" yesterday, which is spot on. It sometimes goes against the grain of "serious" martial artists but when used correctly is a very important aspect of the learning process. This kind of atmosphere helps unlock people's creativity. I think Andy mentioned something about being guided / allowed to explore the work rather than have someone tell you what to do all the time. It doesn't mean the work is any less serious but it does drive away an awful lot of the pretension, posing and preening that we sometimes see in martial arts teaching

5. The subject of martial arts politics came up in chat at the end. The overwhelming impression was of just how little interest people take in it. Mark said something along the lines of " the training is good, that's all I'm worried about" and it seems only a minority take much notice of what goes on on Facebook (so they won't see this ha!)

6. I said in the circle at the end – a day of spirited training with various sharp, heavy, pointy objects and there is no blood on the floor. A testament to the care everyone takes with their training partners, but also the fact they are able to take care of themselves as well, in terms of monitoring psyche and tension levels. I'm sure health and safety would have a fit.... but it shows you can work up to intense levels without damaging each other

7. Development. It's plain to see how much the regulars have developed this year – in fact some of them have become instructors themselves! This is the bottom line for me – results. Nothing else really matters. What people say, what they think.... what matters is the results we get through our training. Not just on a "fighty" level but in all aspects of life. Results have been good and I put it down to two things – the hard work of the people involved and the training methods we use, for which the credit goes to my teachers. Contrary to what some say we don't "add in" combatives or parkour or "structure breaking" or anything else. It's all there, sometimes you just have to work a bit to find it. But that work itself is part of the process, part of the method to unlock your own individuality and creativity. In martial arts it's the easiest thing in the world to knock out little clones of yourself. It's also soul destroying, boring and at the end of the day a waste of everyone's time and money.

8. Lastly and by no means leastly......we found out just how dangerous a coconut can be in the right hands.... who'd have thought!

Thanks everyone for a great day and a great year's training!

RESOURCES

Systema HQ Moscow	www.systemaryabko.com
Systema HQ Toronto	www.russianmartialart.com
Cutting Edge Systema	www.systemauk.com
E-mail	systemauk@outlook.com
Systema books & Instructional films	www.systemafilms.com
General health books and films	www.simplyflow.myshopify.com
Health training	www.simplyflow.co.uk
Tommy Floyd, Florida Systema	www.systemafloyd.com

RECOMMENDED READING

Strikes - Vladimir Vasiliev & Scott Meredith

Let Every Breath - Vladimir Vasiliev

Secrets of the Russian Blade Masters - Vladimir Vasiliev

The Systema Manual - Major Konstantin Komarov

Konstantin Komarov Training Children article

www.russianmartialart.com/article_info.php?articles_id=102

Other books by Robert Poyton

Systema Solo Training
Systema Partner Training
Systema Awareness Training
Systema Voices
Systema Locks and Holds
Systema for Seniors
Systema Self Defence
Fitness Over 40
Don't Worry - A Guide to Stress Management
The Eight Brocades Qigong Exercise

www.ingramcontent.com/pod-product-compliance
Lightning Source LLC
Chambersburg PA
CBHW081616100526
44590CB00021B/3465